ЛЕЧЕНИЕ СНОМ
ПРИ НЕВРОЗАХ

LECHENIE SNOM PRI NEVROZAKH

SLEEP THERAPY IN THE NEUROSES

The

International Behavioral Sciences

Series

editor Joseph Wortis, M.D.

SLEEP THERAPY
IN THE NEUROSES

by

B. V. ANDREEV, M.D.

TRANSLATED FROM RUSSIAN

by Basil Haigh, M.A., M.B., B. Chir.

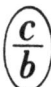

Springer Science+Business Media, LLC

The original Russian text was
published by the Leningrad
branch of Medgiz, the State Press
for Medical Literature, in 1959.

ISBN 978-1-4899-4844-1   ISBN 978-1-4899-4842-7 (eBook)
DOI 10.1007/978-1-4899-4842-7

Library of Congress Catalog Card Number: 60-13947
© 1960 Springer Science+Business Media New York
Originally published by Consultants Bureau Enterprises, Inc in 1960.
Softcover reprint of the hardcover 1st edition 1960

CONTENTS

SLEEP THERAPY
IN THE NEUROSES

This volume was edited during the tenure of a grant MY-2679 from the National Institute of Mental Health for the translation and interpretation of Russian psychiatric literature.

FOREWORD

After a long lifetime of fruitful work Pavlov in the last decade of his career turned his interest to human psychiatric problems. The stimulus for this interest came largely from his observation of conditions in his experimental animals that strikingly resembled human disorders: neurotic disorganization in the face of conflict or stress, partial hysterical paralysis or total catatonic states resulting from fright or exhaustion, and—most interesting of all—a series of abnormal phenomena encountered in animals as they lapsed into drowsiness and sleep. Pavlov was convinced that sleep, hypnosis, and hysteria represented different types and degrees of inhibition, and came to regard certain morbid conditions in both animal and man as reflections of partial inhibitory states. He also concluded that inhibition often develops in response to stress to spare the organism further stimulation and strain. Some individuals, weaker than others, are more prone to retreat into this state of protective or limiting inhibition, and even the healthiest organism, weakened by strain or disease, may be taxed to its limits and lapse into the inhibitory state.

For this weakness, wrote Pavlov, various causes, both hereditary and acquired, may be responsible.... But naturally, when such a nervous system encounters difficulties, more often in a critical physiological and social period of life, it inevitably becomes exhausted after excessive excitation. But exhaustion is one of the chief physiological impulses for the appearance of inhibition in the capacity of a protective process. Hence chronic hypnosis is inhibition in different degrees of extension and intensity. Consequently, this state is, on the one hand, pathological, since it interferes with the patient's normal activity, and, on the other hand, because of its mechanism, it is still physiological, a process of physiological repair, since it protects the cortical cells from the danger of being destroyed as a result of excessive demands.

3

In our laboratory we see striking examples of the way in which prolonged inhibition revives normal activity for a while in weakened cortical cells. There are reasons to assume that as long as the inhibitory process operates, the cortical cells are not gravely damaged, their full return to normal is still possible, they can recover from excessive exhaustion and their pathological process remains reversible. Using modern terminology, it is only a functional disease. . . .*

As a result Pavlov not only recommended an especially quiet sheltered routine for such patients but encouraged the reinforcement of this protective inhibition by the use of sleep. In 1935 he reported a case of catatonic schizophrenia successfully treated by this method. Though sleep treatment had long been used elsewhere, especially in Switzerland, it was Pavlov who provided the theoretical basis for the wide use of sleep treatment in psychiatry in recent years in the Soviet Union.

The knowledge of the healing power of sleep, "that knits up the ravelled sleeve of care," goes back into antiquity, and sleep treatment has been widely used for decades in England, on the Continent, in South America, and—less widely—here. Yet it was S. Weir Mitchell in his "Fat and Blood" who half a century ago gave scientific support and popularity to the term "rest cure" in this country. In the past alcohol, opium, ether, and chloroform had been used to induce sleep, but the synthesis of the barbiturates encouraged the use of new techniques and combinations, with the danger of pneumonia reduced by the concomitant use of antibiotics. Both insulin coma and electronarcosis can be regarded as variants of sleep treatment, and the newer tranquilizing drugs have been used singly and in combination to promote rest and sleep. The use of sleep treatment or protective inhibition has not been limited to psychiatric disorders but has been applied to the treatment of a variety of psychosomatic disorders, especially peptic ulcers, as well as in certain surgical conditions where neural factors are presumably involved.

---

*From Pavlov's article "An Attempt of a Physiologist to Digress into the Domain of Psychiatry," first published in 1930, and available in translation in Pavlov's Selected Works, Moscow, 1955, as well as in Gantt's translation of Pavlov's "Conditioned Reflexes and Psychiatry" New York, 1941.

The Russian experiences should prove to be valuable to the English and American psychiatrist, for the experience is large and varied and has by no means congealed into settled convictions. The first reports of Russian work were based on imported techniques, such as the use of Cloetta's mixture by rectal infusion, described by Richter and Stepanov in 1936, followed soon after by the work of Ivanov-Smolenskii, Yagodka and Ilinskii and others. The barbiturates, especially sodium amytal, soon succeeded other drugs, electronarcosis still enjoys a vogue, but the latest emphasis in the Soviet literature has been on the desirability of inducing drugless natural sleep. Even the earliest workers appreciated the importance of psychological factors and of psychotherapy in managing this treatment and, as Dr. Andreev emphasizes, psychic trauma, unresolved conflicts and disturbing thoughts can vitiate the effects of sleep treatment if these psychological factors are neglected.

Dr. Andreev makes clear that the use of sleep treatment is far from a panacea, and he correctly complains of the over-enthusiastic excesses which threatened to discredit an essentially useful tool in the psychiatric armamentarium. What recommends this book especially is his cautious and discriminating effort to find appropriate indications for the treatment and to elaborate safe and controllable techniques for its application.

The book should serve not only to encourage the use of a valuable form of treatment, but should help to point up the importance of a type of clinical approach and analysis that can relieve and refine the raw empiricism upon which so much current psychiatric treatment is still forced to depend.

JOSEPH WORTIS, M.D.
N. Y. State University
Downstate Medical Center
Brooklyn, N. Y.

INTRODUCTION

Modern sleep therapy is based on Pavlov's concept of protective or restorative inhibition and on the findings of cortico-visceral physiology and pathology. The historical development of this method of treatment can be briefly sketched. The first, or pre-Pavlovian period was characterized by the haphazard empirical use of deep sleep, induced by narcotics, for states of excitement encountered in psychiatric practice. As our knowledge of higher nervous activity increased, sleep therapy began to be used in 1936, during Pavlov's lifetime, in psychiatric practice on a new pathophysiological basis, for the purpose of strengthening the natural protective inhibition. Although narcotics continued to be used for the induction of sleep, they were gradually replaced by sedatives, in doses which did not induce such severe toxic effects and which, moreover, avoided the risk of fatalities.

Some workers (Asratyan, 1954; Stepanskii, 1953) concluded from their own research that in certain pathological conditions the best therapeutic results were obtained from a drug-induced sleep which closely resembled natural sleep, whereas the profound sleep induced by narcotics sometimes even aggravated the pathological process.

The method of sleep therapy gradually emerged from the psychiatric clinic and began to find application in neuroses, in pathological conditions of cortico-visceral origin (hypertension and peptic ulcer), and in many other diseases. Under the direction of B. N. Birman, the Pavlov Clinic for Nervous Diseases was one of the first centers in which sleep therapy, without toxic effect, was used in the treatment of neuroses. The use of this method of treatment was especially advocated after the Joint Session of the two Academies (1950). Unfortunately, enthusiasm for the method was associated with a certain amount of popularization; its widespread abuse, in complete disregard of proper indications, led to a reduction, and sometimes complete elimination, of any therapeutic effect. Ivanov-Smolenskii (1951) warned against the irresponsible spread of the use of sleep therapy and against its misapplication as a panacea. Meanwhile experimental findings on animals showed that drug-induced sleep did not always have a beneficial effect on pathological processes, but sometimes aggravated their course (Galkin, 1953; Stepanskii, 1953; Zdrodovskii, 1953; Uchitel', 1954).

Sleep therapy has been the topic of discussion of many conferences. Whereas at the Ryazan conference in 1952 nearly all the speakers acclaimed the effectiveness of sleep therapy, at the Moscow conference in 1954 a series of papers were presented describing experimental work which demonstrated the adverse effects of hypnotic drugs (and, in particular, of sodium amytal) on the body, and especially on the central nervous system. The unfavorable effect of drug-induced sleep on the course of certain infectious diseases in animals was also described. Work which was reported at the last conference in Tartu in 1955, however, aimed at a deeper elucidation of the mechanisms of the physiological action of therapeutic sleep, and the importance of further study of the problems of treatment by protective inhibition was recognized.

The author of this book has set himself the aim of summarizing the extensive experience gained by himself and by other research workers on sleep therapy. The material for the book has been collected since 1946 in the nervous diseases division (Pavlov Clinic for Nervous Diseases) of the I. P. Pavlov Institute of Physiology of the Academy of Sciences of the USSR. The first director of this clinic was Professor B. N. Birman and its present head is Professor N. A. Kryshova[1]. Experimental research was carried out by the author in the Laboratory of the Physiology and Pathology of Higher Nervous Activity (Chief: Professor F. P. Maiorov).

When the sleep therapy method was introduced in certain hospitals, toxic manifestations were sometimes observed after the use of large doses of sedatives. We have avoided using such large doses, because we felt that the development of unaccustomed and distressing sensations, especially in neurotic patients, could

---

[1]The Pavlov Clinic for Nervous Diseases was organized in 1931, when it was located in the Neuropsychiatric Hospital of the Sverdlovsk district of Leningrad, and was transferred in 1957 to the I. P. Pavlov Clinical Psychoneurological Hospital.

impede recovery. Our efforts were concentrated on the creation of appropriate conditions and the use of the proper influences to strengthen the natural protective inhibition, by prolonging sleep in a form approximating the physiological. We have therefore dwelt in detail on the study of possible ways of producing and utilizing conditioned reflex sleep, in which sedative drugs are replaced by inert substances. In an attempt to produce sleep without toxic manifestations we have also used hypnosis, suggestion, and certain physical sleep-inducing stimuli, as a result of which the dosage of hypnotic drugs has been reduced to a minimum. This method of treatment has been found quite effective and has eliminated the side-effects due to sedatives.

In the assessment of the duration of therapeutic sleep we have employed the objective method of actography, recording the motor activity of the subject, which in most cases allows us accurately to record the transition from waking to sleep and vice versa. By the use of this method we were able to make observations on the efficacy of various measures in prolonging sleep. We have improved the technique of actography and have adapted it to clinical practice. The main advantages of this method are that the motor activity is recorded automatically, without the intervention of the experimenter, continuously for 24 hours, and the subject's sleep is not disturbed.

In a proportion of patients the higher nervous activity was investigated by experimental methods, which served as a valuable supplement to the clinical observations when the course of the patient's condition was being studied.

When using sleep therapy we did not exclude other forms of treatment, but on the contrary we considered that the treatment could be most effective only in combination with other influences acting on the patient. After the conclusion of the course of sleep therapy, we continued to use psychotherapy in various forms, to rehabilitate weakened functions, etc.

As a result of the action of therapeutic sleep the tonus of the cerebral cortex was increased, and on this background the subsequent therapeutic measures brought the treatment to a successful conclusion.

MODERN VIEWS ON NEUROSES

The development of Pavlov's teaching marked the turning point at which the established ideas of the whole of medicine began to be revised. The theory of "nervism" based on his concept of higher nervous activity was developed experimentally, and a new understanding was gained of neuroses and psychoses; the pathophysiological mechanisms of their symptomatology and syndromes began to be studied. The new ideas began to be widely used in practice, especially after the Joint Session of the Academy of Medical Sciences of the USSR in 1950 and after the Special Session in 1952 devoted to the state of neurology and psychiatry.

The Pavlovian view of neuroses has been dealt with adequately in special studies (Birman, 1939, 1951, 1951a; Ivanov-Smolenskii, 1949, and others), and we shall therefore dwell only briefly on a few points which in our opinion merit particular attention.

In the Pavlovian view a neurosis is a functional disorder of the higher nervous activity brought about by functional means, i.e., by presenting the nervous system with tasks beyond its powers (Birman, 1939). In man this functional factor is psychogenic; in some cases, however, a somatic agent is also present, which creates a favorable soil for the development of a neurosis, as Davidenkov (1952), Myasishchev (1955), and others have indicated. Overfatigue, chronic lack of sleep, infections, the menopause, and trauma, any of these can weaken the nervous system, and against this background even the slightest psychogenic factors (social or family conflicts) can produce a neurosis. On the other hand, a complicated situation of conflict can operate for a long time without producing a disease, but the addition of any one of the above somatic factors may provoke a neurotic reaction to preexisting difficulties. Ivanov-Smolenskii (1949) wrote that neuroses are probably more often than not the result of the combined action of both psychogenic and somatogenic traumata. Research by Pervov (1957) showed that in more than half the cases of neurosis which he investigated (55 of 97 cases) the onset was due to the combined action of psychogenic and somatogenic factors.

Pavlov found that a neurosis often developed on the basis of a nervous system of a weak and unbalanced type. A neurosis may arise however even in persons with a strong and balanced nervous system as the result of more severe life experiences, or as a result of trauma, infection, or toxic influences. The material collected by ourselves (1956) and by Pervov (1957) fully supports this view.

Pavlov divided the whole gamut of the various neuroses into three main forms: neurasthenia, hysteria, and psychasthenia, the characteristics of which may be represented in the form of the following scheme.

Scheme of the Main Neuroses

Name of neuroses	Characteristics of the main pathophysiological mechanisms	Forms of the neuroses
Neurasthenia	Pathological weakness or imbalance of nervous processes with balanced primary and secondary signal systems	a) Excitatory (with relative preponderance of the process of excitation) b) Asthenic, or depressive (with weakness of both processes—different phases of overflow inhibition) c) Cyclic (with periodic alteration of a state of increased capacity for work and depression in a strong, excitable type)
Hysteria	Pathological predominance of the primary signal system and subcortex over the secondary signal system in a weak (more rarely in a strong) general type*	a) In a weak type b) In a strong type†
Psychasthenia	Pathological predominance of the secondary signal system over the first and the subcortex in a weak general type	None distinguished

*Relative predominance of the primary signal system and subcortex is understood.
†F. P. Maiorov (1946): S. N. Davidenkov (1957).

Pavlov provided a pathophysiological framework for the concept of neurosis, indicated the general outlines of a classification of the neuroses, distinguished the three main forms, and determined methods of treatment. Does this mean that the problem of the neuroses has now been finally solved? Although Pavlov's main views on neuroses are still regarded as true today, there are differences of opinion on certain details.

We must consider, in particular, the neurosis or syndrome of the obsessive states. An obsessive state may be encountered in various diseases [neuroses, manic-depressive psychosis, schizophrenia, epilepsy, and organic diseases of the brain (Ozeretskovskii, 1950)].

The obsessive state syndrome is often encountered in psychasthenia, and for this reason these two states were previously regarded as identical. Pavlov gave his own clear interpretation of psychasthenia, and considered "obsessive neurosis" separately (Pavlov, 1949, Pavlov's Wednesdays, Vol. 1, p. 342; Pavlov's Wednesday Clinics, pp. 248–249). Although Pavlov used the term "obsessive neurosis" and gave a pathophysiological analysis of this condition, he also accepted the existence of an obsessive syndrome in various neuroses.

Gakkel' (1956) and Dotsenko (1953) regard obsession as a syndrome. A group of authors, among them Ivanov-Smolenskii and his co-workers (Ivanov-Smolenskii, 1955; Seredina, 1955, and others) often use the term "neurosis of obsessive states."

There is thus no general agreement yet on whether the neurosis of the obsessive states should be distinguished as a separate nosological form or regarded as a syndrome.

Our experience has led us to regard the majority of obsessions as a syndrome, making an exception of those rare cases where the obsessions form the essential core of the neurosis.

Some authors include in the term neurosis obsessive states and the various phobias, although Pavlov had previously indicated the different pathophysiological mechanism of the obsessions and impulses, on the one hand, and of the phobias on the other. Whereas he regarded the first two forms as mainly the result of a pathological inertia or stasis of the process of excitation, he regarded phobias as a pathological condition of inhibition.

Birman (1939), Davidenkov (1952), and others supported this differential approach to the obsessions. Belousova (1954) showed that phobias and obsessions unconnected with fear differed from each other in respect to their origin, the state of the higher nervous activity, and the results of sleep therapy.

It is not always possible to encompass the whole diversity of neurotic manifestations in one single diagnosis, for example, neurasthenia, hysteria, and so on. In our clinic we therefore use expanded diagnoses, indicating the more prominent manifestations or syndrome of a particular neurosis. The syndromes most frequently found in practice are: 1) astheno-depressive, 2) syndrome of obsessive states, 3) phobic, 4) fear syndrome[1], 5) hypochondriac, 6) syndrome of visceral disturbances (affecting the cardiovascular system, the gastrointestinal tract, respiration, etc.).

In view of the fact that the physical factors often play an essential role in weakening the nervous system and predisposing it to neurosis, we mention these factors when formulating the diagnosis. Examples of expanded diagnoses are: neurasthenia with a cardiophobic syndrome; hysteria with a syndrome of visceral disorder (affecting the gastrointestinal tract) associated with the menopause; neurasthenia with an astheno-depressive syndrome in association with a past history of brain trauma; etc.

PROTECTIVE INHIBITION

Our knowledge of protective inhibition has developed from both clinical observation and laboratory experiments. Pavlov expressed the view that a single pathophysiological mechanism was responsible for the changes in the motor sphere observed in schizophrenia (catatonic stupor, catalepsy), in hypnosis in man, in the transitional stages between waking and sleep encountered in laboratory animal experiments, and finally, in decerebrate animals (catalepsy, tonic reflexes). Pavlov accounted for these phenomena by the exclusion of the motor portion of the cerebral cortex—in the latter case by anatomical means, and otherwise, by functional means; in both cases this leads to a disinhibition

---

[1]We distinguish these two syndromes, associating ourselves with Birman's point of view. In the phobias, the state of fear is usually caused by a definite situation or an object with which it is closely connected. Apart from this situation, the patient feels normal. In the fear syndrome, violent vegetative crises develop from time to time with the state of fear, mainly without any outward motive and arising in various situations. Mixed and transitional states, however, also exist.

of the lower reflex motor mechanisms. This functional exclusion, suppression, or inhibition is temporary and partial in character.

Experimental studies of different phases of the inhibitory state were carried out by the Pavlov school and the limits of working capacity of the cortical cell were investigated. This research led to the gradual emergence and elucidation of the concept of protective inhibition.

By 1930 Pavlov (1949) had elaborated his idea of the role of inhibition as a protection for the cells of the cortex. He concluded that inhibition protects the affected cortical cells of catatonics from countless external stimuli and enables them to preserve a residue of vital activity and to maintain their resistance against noxious influences to avoid destruction.

Pavlov regarded a group of phenomena observed in schizophrenia as hypnotic phases, understanding by this term intermediate phases between waking and complete sleep. These include: the absence of any reaction when the patient is addressed in a loud voice associated with the appearance of a reaction to a whisper (paradoxical phase); negativism, stereotypy and catatonia, which may also be observed in dogs in intermediate states (obvious manifestations of catatonia, developing during a laboratory experiment, were described by Petrova in 1937); echolalia and echopraxia, also encountered in individual cases during hypnosis in healthy persons; silly and kittenish behavior, characteristic of the hebephrenic form of schizophrenia and observed in healthy persons in the first stages of alcoholic intoxication and also in children and puppies before falling asleep. All these phenomena in man and in animals have a common physiological mechanism, namely, they are characterized by the presence of partial inhibition in the cerebral cortex, or of partial sleep.

"After all that has been said," wrote Pavlov, "it can hardly be doubted that schizophrenia, in its known variants and phases, is in fact a chronic hypnosis."[1]

Pavlov thought that the basis "of this hypnosis is a weak nervous system, especially weakness of the cortical cells." Excitation beyond their capacity leads to exhaustion and this, in turn, causes protective inhibition which, "on the one hand is patholog-

---

[1] I. P. Pavlov, "The tentative excursion of a physiologist in the realm of psychiatry. Complete Collected Works, Vol. 3, p. 409, 1949 [in Russian].

ical, for it deprives the patient of the possibility of normal activity, and on the other hand the mechanism is still essentially physiological, for it protects the cortical cells against their threatened destruction by overwork beyond their capacity."[1]

Several later researches of the Pavlov school were devoted to the investigation of limiting inhibition as a form of protective inhibition. Pavlov expounded his concept of limiting inhibition in detail in 1932 in a paper presented at the International Physiological Congress in Rome (1949a). In this paper, Pavlov cited N. E. Vvedenskii's parabiotic theory of inhibition, which the latter had derived from his investigations on the nerve fiber. In the same year, 1932, in another paper, Pavlov placed limiting inhibition in the unconditioned inhibition group (1949b).

Ivanov-Smolenskii (1936) and his co-workers made a detailed study of the manifestations of protective inhibition in schizophrenia and also in other conditions (1935). They showed that the interlocking or coupling function, i.e., the formation of new conditioned motor reflexes, is severely disorganized in catatonics. The inhibition may be local in character, affecting mainly one particular area: the motor-kinesthetic, visual, auditory, or tactile analyzers. Ivanov-Smolenskii also wrote (1936) that local inhibition sometimes has the character of a pathodynamic structure, the reflection in the cerebral cortex of some difficult situation in life, some serious conflict, presenting on some occasion a task straining to the utmost the capacity of the nervous system of the patient and providing a cause for the development of the disease. Here also belong those cases of delirium in which Pavlov saw the expression of an ultraparadoxical phase, i.e., cases where within the confines of a particular theme only, the patient begins to show signs of oneiroid, hypnoid delirium, etc.

Protective inhibition in schizophrenia may for a time descend to lower levels of the central nervous system and involve the subcortex. This is shown by disappearance or marked depression of the unconditioned (orienting, food, defensive, etc.) reflexes.

Ivanov-Smolenskii's co-workers also observed inhibition of the unconditioned vegetative reflexes (respiratory and cardiovascular). In many catatonics, stimulation with a faradic current,

---

[1] I. P. Pavlov, Complete Collected Works, Vol. 3, p. 410 [in Russian].

16

even of considerable strength, does not elicit the usual vegetative reactions but, on the contrary, the pulse is often observed to be slowed and the respiratory excursions diminished. In certain rare catatonic cases, there is a loss of voluntary activity and speech, but no gross disturbances of muscle tone, while the unconditioned reactions are acutely intensified and irradiated, taking on the character of diffuse reactions. This is evidently due to positive induction to the subcortex from the inhibited cortex.

The different forms of change in muscle tone in catatonics suggest, according to Ivanov-Smolenskii's findings, a different extent of spread of the inhibition, and moreover in these patients the trend of the changes in muscle tone can not only be observed throughout the duration of the disease but also from day to day, with the onset of nocturnal sleep when the tone passes through the phases of catalepsy, tonic contraction, and flaccid immobility. In schizophrenia, however, the chronic inhibition does not usually attain the degree of deep sleep. The borderline between waking and sleep under these circumstances appears to be obliterated. These patients spend the whole time in a phase intermediate between waking and sleeping.

All the phenomena described are due to temporary inhibition and not to destruction of the cells, for when the patients emerge from their catatonic stupor, these phenomena disappear. The protective inhibition in schizophrenia may also be abolished by abnormal, artificial means. Narbutovich and Golovina (1934), for instance, showed that injection of alcohol in catatonics caused them to become disinhibited, so that they once more resumed contact, regained the power of speech, etc., but when the protective inhibition reappeared later it was stronger and reached a greater depth, and the patients fell into a deep sleep.

The manifestations of protective inhibition have recently been studied in conditions other than schizophrenia. The course of regression of the profound protective limiting inhibition appearing immediately after epileptic fits (Seredina, 1941) and after convulsions in schizophrenics induced by cardiazol and electric shock (Gartsshtein, 1940; Traugott, 1957) has been carefully studied.

In a series of experimental investigations, Gartsshtein (1951, 1952, 1953) showed the presence of manifestations of protective limiting inhibition, manifested in various degrees or phases involving both the primary and secondary signal systems, in the reactive depressions. After sleep therapy the nervous system was strengthened and the signs of protective inhibition diminished and disappeared.

Fadeeva (1947) investigated the reasons why, in cyclothymia, as the manic state develops more strongly, there is a gradual increase in the manifestations of limiting protective inhibition, at first affecting the highest and complex forms of activity of the secondary signal system (the higher associations), then the more primitive forms, and finally extending also to the primary signal system.

Overflow protective inhibition is very marked in the addictions, particulary in chronic alcoholism. In these patients Strel'-chuk (1949) found some difficulty in the development of conditioned connections, a loss of mobility in the basic nervous processes, and a disturbance of internal inhibition. After prolonged abstinence from alcohol and after suitable treatment cortical activity was revived.

Sinkevich (1951) used a motor-speech method to study patients suffering from chronic alcoholism; replacing the direct stimuli by verbal stimuli, and sometimes observed equivalent (i.e., all reactions equal) and paradoxical phases. The degree to which these were expressed in the primary and secondary signal systems varied in their relative proportions. Following treatment the phasic manifestations diminished or disappeared in both signal systems.

Asratyan (1944, 1948) concerned himself with problems of protective inhibition following injuries to the nervous system. He called this inhibition "remedial protective," and for therapeutic purposes he reinforced it with drug-induced sleep. Asratyan points out that the sequelae of organic lesions of the central and peripheral nervous system are due not only to destruction or injury to the nerve cells or nerve fibers but also to the special functional state—namely protective inhibition—of wide areas of the nervous system not directly involved by the trauma. This phenomenon has long been known under the name of central shock or diaschisis. This protective inhibition may lead to the disappearance of certain reflexes and the onset of transient palsies or weakness.

Asratyan applied this understanding of the importance of remedial protective inhibition as a post-traumatic biological phenomenon to develop practical therapeutic measures, viz, pharmacological sleep treatment, which proved highly effective both in animal experiments and with human subjects.

Ivanov-Smolenskii and his associates (1951) have done some experimental research on the phenomena of protective inhibition after closed and open brain injuries in man. Studies of a series of successive periods in the regression of protective inhibition in these conditions showed that the lower divisions of the brainstem are the first to be freed from inhibition, then the divisions nearest to the cerebral cortex, and lastly the structures implicated in the secondary signal system.

Deaf-mutism, often observed after concussion from the explosion of a bomb or shell at close quarters, can be regarded with every justification as a manifestation of protective inhibition. In fact one usually cannot find sufficient localized changes in the nervous system to account for this syndrome. It may also develop without any evidence of brain concussion, i.e., without the direct participation of a physical traumatic agent. Sooner or later this syndrome disappears, in the majority of cases quickly, and sometimes quite unexpectedly. This suggests the functional nature of the condition, which can be regarded as a manifestation of fixed protective inhibition. An analysis of the physiological mechanism of this syndrome has been made by Fedorov (1944). He connected its development with the fact that the tension of the nervous system, and especially of the functions of speech and hearing, was maximal at the moment of injury amidst all the din of the battlefield.

In papers by Birman (1946, 1951) a detailed analysis is made of neurotic syndromes from the point of view of the concept of protective inhibition. It now became possible to regard the various symptoms encountered in all three main forms of neurosis— neurasthenia, hysteria, and psychasthenia—as expressions of protective inhibition. This may assume demonstrable form, for example, a stuporous or cataleptic state following an emotional shock, or a hysterical hypnotic state or reactive sleep following some unpleasant experiences, but it may also be masked. The fact that a patient is apparently awake should not deceive us, says Birman, for all variations and degrees of the hypnotic state can be encountered, ranging from scarcely detectable conditions to complete sleep.

Pavlov concluded that a person suffering from hysteria "may and must appear chronically hypnotized to some degree, even in the ordinary conditions of life, for in the presence of cortical weakness, even ordinary stimuli must be supramaximal and the overflow leads to limiting inhibition. . ." (1949b, p. 473). Such hysterical symptoms as anesthesia, paralysis, and mutism are the result of a dissociation of cortical activity involving partial or hypnotic inhibition. The enhanced emotionality and impressionability of hysterical subjects are due to the state of inhibition of the secondary signal system, with disinhibition of the primary signal system and subcortex.

The characteristic loss by the psychasthenic of his sensation of reality, the sensation that actual events seem like phantasies and dreams, all this was regarded by Birman (1951) as a manifestation of the parabiotic phase of inhibition, in which external stimuli, impinging on the weakened primary signal system of the psychasthenic, become overwhelming and induce only a weak effect. No dissociation of cortical activity is observed in psychasthenia, however, because the secondary signal system, as the higher level of integrative activity of the nervous system, is affected less here than in the hysteric.

A number of functional disturbances in neurasthenia (loss of capacity for mental work, rapid fatiguability, absent-mindedness, apathy) may be explained by the development of protective inhibition. Symptoms of ambivalence, such as, for example, the religiosity with obsessions of a blasphemous character[1] encountered in psychasthenia as well as other forms of neurosis, were attributed by Pavlov to the ultraparadoxical phase of the developing inhibition.

There is no doubt that the disturbances of vegetative function encountered in the neuroses are due to the irradiation of inhi-

---

[1]Nowadays ambivalence more often has a different content; e.g., the love of a child is accompanied by a simultaneous obsessive desire to cause it harm, etc.

bition from the cortex to the subcortical centers or to disinhibition of these centers by the law of positive induction, and are generally the result of disturbance of the regulatory function of the partially inhibited cortex. Platonov (1947) interprets a number of neurotic symptoms in the same way, regarding them as manifestations of hypnoid phases.

The question arises: can any form of inhibition be regarded as protective, or is this property peculiar to limiting (or ultramaximal) inhibition? Pavlov emphasized that inhibition is a process which not only brings to a halt the activity involving tissue damage, but also encourages its repair. Ivanov-Smolenskii says that Pavlov regarded only limiting inhibition as protective, employing the term "protective limiting" inhibition (1951).

Asratyan (1955) believes that there is no special form of inhibition that can be called protective-restorative, but that there is a basic single type of inhibition, active in nature, which has protective-restorative and coordinating properties. The primitive role of inhibition is both protective and restorative, and the coordinating role is a subsequent development in the course of phylogenesis and ontogenesis. Stepanskii (1955) takes the view that all forms of inhibition developing in the central nervous system have protective properties.

Fol'bort and his co-workers (1946) showed experimentally that the application of a differential stimulus at a time when the salivary gland was becoming exhausted after the repeated application of a conditioned stimulus causes an increase in the concentration of the residual solids of the saliva in the subsequent conditioned reflex. This fact thus confirms Pavlov's view that inhibition is a process which not only terminates activity but also promotes restoration, and this moreover shows that coordinating inhibition also is restorative in character—not always, but when some degree of exhaustion is present.

Pavlov repeatedly stressed that imminent functional destruction is the main factor causing the appearance in the nerve cell of inhibition. This inhibition exerts a protective function, by developing before the onset of fatigue and preventing further damage to the cell, which might be dangerous; furthermore, it promotes restoration of the normal composition of the cell.

Fol'bort raises some new questions on this matter. Can the connection between the process of exhaustion and the process of inhibition be broken, he asks, and he cites a case where the connection between these processes is ruptured and exhaustion ceases to be a factor inducing inhibition, and where the least degree of excitation is no longer terminated by inhibition. Examples of this can be found in cases of the so-called excitatory form of shock encountered in war conditions. This form is the most dangerous, for the intensive excitation is not arrested by any process of inhibition, but is only brought to an end by the total exhaustion of the nervous system and, in most cases, by death of the patient. By way of a second example, Fol'bort cites the major epileptic fit. Here, too, inhibition does not develop at the proper time, and the convulsive attack is arrested only after the onset of complete exhaustion of the central nervous system, evidence of which is furnished by the epileptic coma and deep sleep which follow the fit.

The second question posed by Fol'bort concerns the connection between inhibition and recovery. He believes that the two are by no means synonymous, and that inhibition is not always accompanied by recovery. As an example, he cites Kachalkin's catatonic, who remained in a state of deep inhibition for more than 20 years but did not subsequently recover. It is obvious that in this case protective inhibition took place in the sense of prevention of further damage to the nervous system, but not in the sense of recovery. Fol'bort considers that this phenomenon is one further mechanism in the pathology of higher nervous activity, accounting for the development of certain abnormal reactions.

According to Fol'bort, cases of breakdown of the connection between exhaustion and inhibition are seen quite rarely; these are serious pathological conditions, carrying the threat of catastrophe. The breakdown of the connection between inhibition and recovery is not such a rare event and is less dangerous, for here, even if recovery does not take place, the protective role still remains, preventing further fatal damage to the cells.

The concept of protective inhibition, first advanced by Pavlov on the basis of laboratory experiments and the study of schizophrenia, was thus subsequently used to explain many of the symptoms observed in psychoneuroses. It has been shown that many pathological phenomena are due, not to disturbances of the structure of nerve tissues, but to temporary inhibition, protective in character. This provided a new approach to the treatment of patients presenting these phenomena, and therapeutic measures began to be used which were aimed at strengthening the protective inhibition, particularly sleep therapy.

A BRIEF OUTLINE OF THE HISTORY OF
THE METHOD OF SLEEP THERAPY

The empirical use of narcotic sleep as a method of treatment in psychiatric practice was described as long ago as the middle of the nineteenth century, but it became much more widespread in the twenties and thirties of the present century (Ivanov-Smolenskii, 1940, and others). In the West this method of treatment, remained empirical for a long time and was used mainly in a variety of pathological conditions characterized by a generalized motor excitation which remained resistant to ordinary sedative measures, e.g., in schizophrenia associated with insomnia, excitation, or hallucinations, and in some other psychoses. This treatment amounted to a prolongéd general anesthesia, was accompanied by somatic complications (mainly affecting the cardiovascular and respiratory systems) and, because of this, was marked by a high mortality rate (Ivanov-Smolenskii, 1951).

The use of narcotic sleep by a number of psychiatrists in the USSR began in the 1930's (Protopopov, 1937; Shevelev, 1936; Gilyarovskii, 1936; Landkof, 1938; Rikhter, 1937; Sereiskii, 1937; and others). However, not all of them were guided by the Pavlovian principle of protective inhibition, but rather by the experiences and the interpretations of the mechanism of the treatment brought out by foreign psychiatrists.

The first attempt to use therapeutic sleep as a method of psychiatric therapy (in schizophrenia), based on pathogenic concepts, was carried out at Pavlov's suggestion, because of his views on schizophrenia, and took place at the Pavlov Psychiatric Clinic under the direction of Ivanov-Smolenskii in 1936. The results were encouraging and gratifying to Pavlov himself, by confirming the correctness of his concept and opening new prospects for the use of this method of treatment.

Ivanov-Smolenskii (1937, 1938, 1939, 1951) regarded the pathophysiological mechanism of the therapeutic action of prolonged narcosis in the psychoses as a combination of two closely related factors: a passive defensive component (protective inhibition) and an active defensive component (vegetative self-defense). Approximately the same view was held by other authors (Gilyarovskii, Sereiskii, Shevelev), although they attached greater importance to the second factor—stimulation (Reiztherapie)—while the sleep factor itself was relegated to a subordinate position, since during prolonged narcosis intensive endogenous protein destruction, blood picture changes, and "vegetative mobilization" occur, and patients who slept for only a few hours improved as much as those who slept for longer periods.

Some of the authors cited above thought that the therapeutic action of prolonged narcosis in the psychoses depended also on the special state of the patient after arousal, when his helplessness and the "mellowing" of his psyche made him amenable to psychotherapy. Protopopov criticized this interpretation of the therapeutic action of prolonged narcosis put forth by foreign authors, and felt that the main therapeutic factor was the protective inhibition.

After five years experience with narcotic sleep therapy at the Pavlov Psychiatric Clinic, certain improvements were made in the technique of treatment (Ivanov-Smolenskii, 1951). Cloetta's mixture, and the deep narcosis it induced, were given up because of the severe toxic manifestations and occasional somatic complications. Sodium amytal began to be used, sometimes in combination with paraldehyde or chloral hydrate, in order to produce, not a narcosis, but a prolonged deep sleep lasting 6 to 8 days, and more closely resembling natural physiological sleep. In order to produce vegetative mobilization and, in schizophrenia, to remove those abnormal vegetative metabolic disturbances that were the source of pathological, mainly toxic, influences affecting the higher divisions of the brain, sleep treatment was combined with other active therapeutic methods: sulfosin, insulin (not enough to induce coma), convulsive therapy, etc. (Narbutovich and Y. Pavorinskii, 1939; Yapontsev, 1939; Povorinskii, 1953).

Nevertheless, in spite of the complete abandonment of the use of Cloetta's mixture and the extensive use at the present time of sodium amytal, many psychiatrists have continued until recently to use fairly toxic forms of therapy, producing a sleep differing considerably from the physiological variety.

Chalisov (1939) and Shpir (1939) concluded from their observations that the treatment of schizophrenia was based not on sleep itself, but on the toxicosis, which led to a biological reorganization of the body, as a result of which improvement took place in certain cases. Sleep therapy with large doses of hypnotic drugs, with the development of toxic manifestations, was also used by several other authors in psychiatric hospital practice.

Many psychiatrists, however—Kerbikov et al. (1951), Kokin et al. (1951), Galenko (1953), Rasin and Vernikova (1952), Sereiskii et al. (1953), Shpak (1952), and Lukina (1953)—attempted to reduce the dosage and to use methods of sleep therapy in which toxic effects were eliminated (electro-sleep, conditioned-reflex sleep, hypnosis, etc.) or minimized (by administration of a mixture containing alcohol, barbiturates, and thiamin or glutamic acid, etc.). Naumova (1947) showed that smaller doses of sedatives were needed to produce sleep in schizophrenics than in a control group.

There is as yet no agreement on the mechanism of action of therapeutic sleep in psychic disorders, and especially in schizophrenia. The question arises here, is it only the protective inhibition, in the form of deep sleep, that is of decisive importance, or is it the drug itself, and its toxic properties. Rikhter (1956) in reviewing the data and views of other psychiatrists (Ivanov-Smolenskii, Gilyarovskii, Povorinskii, and others) as well as his own observations over many years, concludes that it is the deep, uninterrupted therapeutic sleep, associated with metabolic changes and reorganization of the entire body, that is of value in schizophrenia. Rikhter attributes the failure of sleep therapy in schizophrenia in the hands of some authors to their use of superficial interrupted sleep, a modality which is indicated in various neuroses and in some psychoses with less pronounced disturbances than in schizophrenia.

Tatarenko (1956), in one of his latest papers, develops the idea of a differential approach to the sleep therapy of schizophrenia. Depending on the stage and pathophysiological picture, in some cases protective therapy in the form of deep sleep is indicated, and in others the use of various forms of active therapy, even to the extent of the induction of isolated electric convulsions.

We have described briefly the current opinions on the mechanism of action of therapeutic sleep in schizophrenia, for it was with this disease that this method of treatment began to be used on pathogenetic grounds. Nowadays sleep therapy has become widely accepted and incorporated in the therapeutic armamentarium of many different clinics. Sleep therapy is effective in various conditions in which patients show marked manifestations of protective inhibition.

THE INDICATIONS FOR SLEEP THERAPY
IN NEUROSES

We have indicated above that the mechanism of protective inhibition lies at the basis of many of the symptoms and syndromes of the neuroses. As Birman wrote, these findings, indicating the great importance of protective inhibition in determining the development and clinical course of the neuroses, were the starting point of research into the treatment of neurosis by sleep and by hypnotic inhibition. The method of sleep therapy, as it developed in psychiatric practice, was thus applied to the neuroses, and was first employed at the Pavlov Clinic for Neuroses in the postwar period (Birman, 1946, 1950, 1951).

At that time the indications for sleep therapy had increased abnormally for various reasons. Many people had been exposed to multiple traumatic experiences during the war (malnutrition, psychic trauma, overstrain), which weakened their nervous and somatic tone. The war left wounds which for a long time continued to inflict trauma on the nervous systems of a certain proportion of the population, disrupting living conditions and family life. In the face of all the special conditions prevailing at that time in the neurotic disorders that were then encountered, it was necessary in the first place to proceed along the lines of strengthening the protective inhibition, by means of sleep therapy and passive psychotherapy (hypnosis and suggestion), in order to restore the working capacity of the exhausted nerve cells, and then subsequently, where necessary, to resort to active psychotherapy. Birman has drawn attention to these considerations (1950, 1951).

In summarizing the experience of our clinic on indications for sleep therapy, Birman wrote (1951) that when a reactive neurotic syndrome arises as a result of noxious influences producing an exhaustion of a relatively intact nervous system, this constitutes an absolute indication for sleep therapy. These neurotic syndromes include anxiety neuroses with vegetative disturbances, reactive phobic syndromes, and psychogenic visceral disturbances. So far as the prolonged chronic, so-called "constitutional" forms of neurosis and neurotic development are concerned, Birman pointed out that in these forms the self-defensive inhibitory reaction is always readily elicited. The main therapeutic agent here was active psychotherapy; in cases with severe asthenia, however, usually observed during a relapse of the neurosis, it was sometimes necessary to administer a course of sleep therapy in order to raise the tone and to create an optimal basis for the subsequent therapeutic measures, namely, active psychotherapy and training.

Most of the authors who use sleep therapy think that, of all the various neurotic conditions, the best therapeutic results are attained in neurasthenia and neurasthenic states, especially in those with an asthenic symptomatology (Davidenkov, 1951; Aleksandrova and Prokhorova, 1953; Kamyanov, 1952; Vaflin, 1952; Kurilenko, 1952; Zaretskii, 1953; Mukhin, 1953; Ostrovskii, 1953; Ershov, 1954; Ivanov, 1955; Sennikov, 1956; and others).

There are some differences of opinion on the value of sleep therapy in hysteria. In general it can be said that the results are not as good as in neurasthenia. For this reason we are very discriminating in our selection of hysterical patients for sleep therapy. Sleep therapy is evidently indicated in those cases where we are dealing with an asthenia of some neurophysiological origin.

Davidenkov (1951) reports good results with sleep therapy in the treatment of hysterical patients, and in these cases he attaches considerable importance to the contribution of psychotherapy. In a series of 8 cases, only one of his patients failed to improve (hysterical syndrome on a background of preexisting concussion); symptoms such as astasia-abasia, hysterical fits, and writer's cramp all disappeared.

On the subject of psychasthenia, the authors mentioned above cite only a small number of cases, which suggests that sleep therapy is of little value in this condition.

The following considerations relate to the value of sleep therapy in various syndromes. It is generally agreed that reactive states respond well to the treatment. Birman observed good results in the anxiety neuroses. Davidenkov (1951, 1953, 1955) had satisfactory results in anxiety syndromes and phobias. According to a number of workers, sleep therapy induces remission in patients with writer's cramp. Of 6 patients with writer's cramp Druzhinin (1953) reported that 4 were cured and 2 improved. Aleksandrova and Prokhorova observed satisfactory results in 7 of 11 cases of writer's cramp. Kondratenko (1953) made a special study of sleep therapy in patients with various forms of writer's cramp, and after a course of sleep he invariably carried out re-education or training. Of his 16 patients, only in 3 was the condition unchanged (the same as in patients who were not given training). This author observes that these two methods (sleep and training), when given separately, do not produce any significant improvement.

There are differences of opinion on the effectiveness of sleep therapy in obsessional states. At a conference on sleep therapy held in Ryazan in 1953 (Extended Meeting, 1953), Strel'chuk declared that these conditions responded well to treatment. Gakkel', on the basis of his own experience, held the opposite opinion. Davidenkov and his associates (1955) believe that obsessional states may be an indication for the use of sleep therapy. In a series of cases described by Davidenkov, most of those who responded to sleep therapy were suffering from phobias; the results were not so good in patients with compulsions and obsessional ideas. These authors point out that improvement was often not seen immediately, but developed during the succeeding month; in only 3 of 17 patients was absolutely no effect observed. Druzhinin reports that, of 17 patients with obsessional states, improvement or recovery was observed in 11. Aleksandrova and Prokhorova got good results in all 9 patients with hysterical hyperkinesis treated with sleep. In 8 of 9 patients with compulsive habits, however, the condition remained unchanged.

The differences of opinion and the doubts regarding the effectiveness of sleep therapy in obsessional states are evidently due to the inclusion of heterogeneous diseases in this group. As we have already remarked, it is necessary to differentiate between anxiety states and obsessional states, which are based on inert foci of excitation (obsessions, compulsions). It will then be found that the former respond well to sleep therapy, but this treatment is less effective in the latter. The same conclusion was reached by Belousova (1954).

If we examine the indications for sleep therapy from the point of view of the characteristics and interrelationships of the fundamental nervous processes, we find that all authors agree that better results are obtained in asthenic or asthenic-depressive forms of neurasthenia than in excitatory forms. Many authors also recommend sleep therapy in asthenic states of different origin, those resulting from brain trauma, infection, toxic agents, etc. (Aleksandrova and Prokhorova). Ivanov reports that, of 26 patients suffering from an asthenic condition, only 3 showed minimal improvement, while the treatment was moderately effective in the rest. Good results were obtained in patients with postinfectious asthenia. Good results were also observed in asthenic states by Solovei (1953).

Birman reported the successful treatment of patients with psychogenic visceral disturbances in our clinic in 1946 and 1950. The use of sleep therapy in typical cortico-visceral diseases, such as hypertension and peptic ulcers, is fairly widespread at the present time. In these diseases, good results have been obtained in cases where the condition had not yet progressed to the stage of serious organic involvement.

Data on the results of sleep therapy in patients with a hypochondriacal syndrome are very scanty. Druzhinin reports that no significant improvement was observed in any of 10 such patients. Of 22 patients with reactive hypochondriacal states treated by Ostrovskii, no effect was found in 6 and in 3 cases exacerbations were observed.

It can thus be concluded from a survey of the literature that the conditions where sleep therapy is most definitely indicated are neuroses of acute and subacute onset (reactive neuroses), and among these, the asthenic or asthenic-depressive forms of neurasthenia in particular. These indications may be understood perfectly from the point of view of the pathophysiological mechanism of these conditions. Under the term "asthenic states" we understand cases where not only the inhibitory process but also the more stable excitatory process is weakened, when manifestations of protective limiting inhibition develop and, consequently, the nerve cell is in greatest need of a strengthening of this protective inhibition, i.e., of sleep therapy.

We carried out a preliminary selection of patients for sleep therapy, using the following criteria on first acquaintance with the patients: intolerance of noise, bright light, and social intercourse; longing for peace, quiet, and solitude; desire to remain in bed asleep for a long time. We found these symptoms most often in patients whose recent history showed exhaustion of the nervous system as the result of acute or prolonged psychic trauma, lack of sleep, and so on. Patient Sm-va (case No. 234, 1954), for instance, became ill as the result of a prolonged conflict in her domestic affairs; for the previous six months she had been unable to have any normal rest or sleep; on admission to the clinic she showed greatly increased drowsiness. In patient S-n (case No. 306, 1953) the nervous system was weakened as the result of a psychic trauma during the war. With this as a background, before falling ill she had become involved in a prolonged conflict in connection with her employment. Among other symptoms this patient presented sensitivity to noise and light.

Patient T-na (case No. 890, 1952) suffered from repeated psychic traumata (loss of her family) during the war, and was now confronted with a conflict in connection with her life situation.

Patient L-na (case No. 82, 1954), the director of a school, had worked hard and for long hours for a considerable period of time (since the beginning of the war) with scarcely any rest. In 1946 her husband died; throughout the next 5 years her daughter was seriously ill. She had to carry out a number of professional and social obligations. During vacations she did not rest. Among several neurotic symptoms, she showed a sharp decline in her capacity for work, intolerance to noise, and a longing for quiet. In all those cases where symptoms of this sort were found, the results of sleep therapy were good. In some patients we observed an increased drowsiness and prolonged natural sleep in the first days of their stay in the clinic.

An indispensable precondition for proceeding with sleep therapy was the desire of the patient himself to undergo this form of treatment and his agreement to conform fully to the prescribed regimen. If we found that a patient reacted badly to long periods of rest in bed, or if the patient declared that he felt better when in the society of others, when he was distracted from his own thoughts, and that he preferred to be on the move, then sleep therapy was not prescribed for this patient.

As an example we cite patient M-ko (case No. 320, 1953), female, aged 21 years, with a diagnosis of hysteria with motor conversion features (the production of a hiccup-like sound) and residual manifestations of a virus encephalitis. The patient was characterized by increased emotionalism, excitability, a general lack of self-restraint, and a longing to be in company (preferably male). An attempt was made to carry out sleep therapy, but it had to be discontinued after 5 days because the patient was unwilling to conform to the "sleep program," and average doses of sedatives (a daily dose of 0.3 g of phenobarbital) did not produce adequate sleep.

THE INVESTIGATION OF SLEEP BY
THE METHOD OF ACTOGRAPHY

In looking for a method of investigation of sleep, in 1940 we tried actography, which was first suggested by Szymanski (1914), and a series of preliminary observations demonstrated that it was a suitable method to use. Later we improved the method and carried out investigations of sleep in healthy subjects and, in particular, in patients suffering from neuroses; we also conducted experiments at the Clinic for Organic Diseases of the Nervous System together with E. A. Karapetyan and Ya. M. Kraevskii (Andreev, 1956).

The method consists of the automatic recording of the motor activity of a person lying in bed. Our first investigations showed that in the majority of cases the actogram is an objective record from which conclusions may be drawn about the sleeping and waking states of the subject, and specially designed experimental studies confirmed that these conclusions were correct.

We used the simplest kind of pickup device, requiring no modifications or accessories, easily attached to any bed, which allowed us to place the recording apparatus some distance outside the ward. The device was a rubber ring cushion beneath the mattress, connected by means of a rubber tube to a recording manometer (Fig. 1). The ring is usually put in position uninflated, for the residual air is sufficient for pneumatic transmission of the subject's movements, and only if the oscillations are of low amplitude, as recorded by the pen, is the ring slightly inflated to the desired degree.

We slightly modified the lever with the recording pen on the manometer, by the addition of a bent penholder, which keeps the pen perpendicular to the revolving surface of the drum as it traces the curve, pressing it against the surface by its own weight (Fig. 2). In this way the reliability of the tracing is assured if the drum should revolve in a slightly eccentric manner. To counterbalance the added writing pen, an adjustable counterpoise is secured to the other side of the lever.

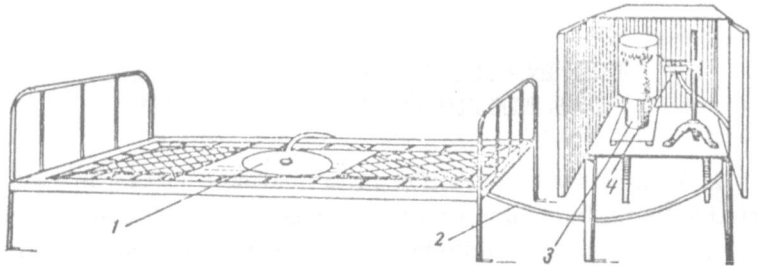

Fig. 1. Scheme of the apparatus for actography. 1) Pickup; 2) rubber tube; 3) clockwork mechanism; 4) Marey's capsule.

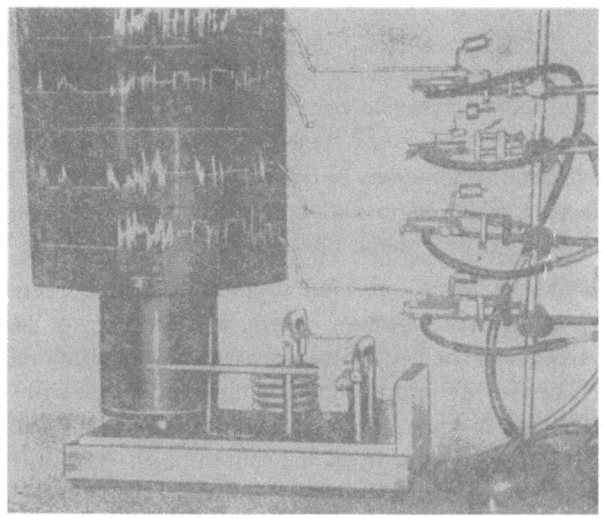

Fig. 2. Recording part of the actographic apparatus. On the left is the revolving drum with actograms, set in motion by the clockwork mechanism (in the lower cylinder) of a barograph. (The remaining details of the mechanism of the barograph are not utilized.) On the right is the stand with the Marey's capsules.

Movement of the drum is powered by a clockwork mechanism providing one complete revolution in 24 hours (from a meteorological apparatus). The ordinary kymograph could not be used here because of its rapid rate of revolution, which would produce

36

a 24-hour actogram of excessive length which could not be scanned at once by the eye, so that it would be impossible to gain an impression of the condition of the subject in the course of the 24 hours. The plastic drum which contains the clockwork mechanism is too small, and therefore, to enlarge the scale of the actogram and to obtain simultaneous tracings from 4 beds, we superimposed on it a cardboard cylinder of greater diameter (20 cm) and a height of 26 cm. The length of the 24-hour actogram is thus 62.4 cm, which is convenient for study; 26 mm is equivalent to 1 hour. Naturally, the length of the actogram may be varied in accordance with the purpose of the investigation and the available technical resources. Berdnik (1955) uses the clockwork mechanism from an alarm clock with a 12-hour period of revolution and traces in ink on a tracing-paper tape winding onto the drum. In order to mark the time (in hours) we apply a rubber stamp with the appropriate lines marked on it and print the figures of the hours on the smoked paper.

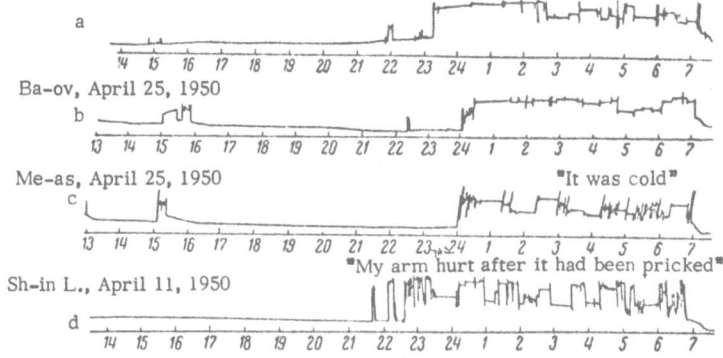

Fig. 3. Actograms of healthy subjects. Legend, top to bottom: actogram, time marker, in hours for 24 hr. The level of the actogram indicates that the subject is no longer on the bed. Actograms a and b indicate sound, peaceful sleep and rapid falling asleep: a) almost instantaneously; b) after 20 minutes. Actograms c and d were obtained during disturbed sleep with frequent awakenings for the reasons indicated on the figure.

Our method enables us to determine whether the subject is awake or asleep, and to estimate to some extent the depth of sleep as reflected in motor activity. Compared with other methods of recording changes in this or that function during the development of sleep, this method possesses many advantages. The more important of these are: 1) the investigation does not disturb the subject's sleep; 2) the experimenter does not need to be present (the recording is automatic); 3) actograms from several beds can be recorded simultaneously; 4) the recording may be continued for many days in order to ascertain the sleep pattern of the subject; 5) the entire apparatus is simple and inexpensive.

This method, however, like many others, is limited to the investigation of only one predetermined function, in this case the motor activity during sleep and waking. In this respect, actography must not be regarded as a substitute for other methods. They may all be employed in the comprehensive study of processes taking place in the intact subject.

It will be seen from the actogram (Fig. 3) that waking is characterized by frequent, almost uninterrupted movements. During sleep, the number of movements at once decreases, and the smooth line of absolute rest is broken from time to time by single cross lines of movements involving changes in the position of the limbs or head or turning over in bed. We therefore usually counted the duration of diurnal and nocturnal sleep in hours and minutes, and added these figures to obtain the total length of sleep in the 24 hours (Fig. 4). These results are transferred to a specially printed form.

Occasionally cases are encountered in which the change from waking to sleep and vice versa are less obvious. We then try to discover the individual peculiarities in the form of the actogram for the person concerned by comparing the curve with the results of interrogation of that person, with information obtained from surrounding persons, and with various events taking place in the course of the 24 hours, in order to establish the actual time of sleeping and waking for this subject. When such a comparison has been made for 2–3 days, we are in a position to define the qualitative characteristics of the actogram which are peculiar to that subject, and we can then "read" the actogram correctly. It is only in cases in which it is difficult to demarcate by means of the actogram the borderline between the states of waking and sleeping, because of the distinctive features of the sleep itself that special treatment of the actogram has to be undertaken. In such patients the dynamics of sleep may be observed for several days, taking as a criterion of the quality (depth) of sleep the intensity of the motor activity. We then estimate over a certain interval of time, for example during the night, the number of "restful" or "restless" 5-min periods (i.e., those in which there is no movement or where there is movement), by placing on the actogram a sheet of graph paper in which the rulings are at a distance corresponding to intervals of 5 min. The "restful" or "restless" 5-min periods are then converted into percentages of the total number of 5-min periods in this particular interval of time, and this index serves as a basis for comparisons with tracings for other nights.

Ne-n, May 6, 1955

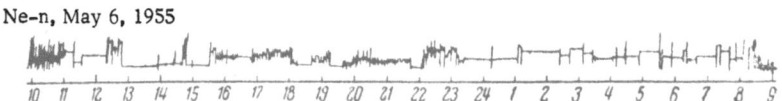

Fig. 4. 24-hour actogram of a patient, on the basis of which a form was compiled for the assessment of sleep. Legend as in Fig. 3.

Investigation of the Duration of Sleep within a 24-Hour Period by the Actographic Method

Surname, and initials   Nenilov, N. B.

Department: III   Date: May 6, 1955

1. Prescription: Phenobarbital 0.05 g morning and evening
2. During the day, slept from 11.00 to 12.20; from 16.25 to 16.45
3. Went to bed at night at   22.05
4. Fell asleep at   23.25
5. Woke up from 5.35 to 5.40   from ___ to ___
6. Got out of bed from 5.35   to 5.40; from ___ to ___
7. Woke up in the morning at 8.15
8. Got up at 9.00

— — — — — — — — — — — — — — — — — — —

   Total no. of hours of sleep: by day   1.40
                                by night 8.45

                                Total: 10.25

   Doctor's signature:

The data obtained over a period of several days on the number of hours of sleep or "restful" 5-min periods is then transferred to graph paper, and the curve of the sleep pattern for this period is constructed. The fluctuations and changes in these indices, depending on the influence of various factors, can then be seen.

Popov (1954) suggests calculating the number of movements during certain intervals of time, for example, half an hour, and on the basis of this, tracing the curve of the pattern of sleep for each night. But some objection may be made to counting the number of movements of a subject with a drum revolving at the rate used, for the strokes are superimposed, and the numbers estimated would be, for this reason, arbitrary. In many cases it is impossible to decide whether to regard a given line as meaning one or several movements. This means that the number of movements counted is relative and subjective. Counting the "restful" or "restless" 5-min intervals, however, is free from these disadvantages. Furthermore, it can hardly be of fundamental importance in determining the character of the sleep if the subject has turned over once or if, in so doing, he has made a few additional movements.

From time to time people with no experience with this method of actography will say that a subject can lie awake, at rest, without movement, so that it is impossible to distinguish between wakefulness and sleep by this means. This is disproved by a demonstration of the facts. Nearly every person, when awake, without realizing it himself performs a large number of different fine movements, which are reflected in the actogram. The intensive motor activity reflects the active state of the brain, i.e., a waking state. Even active inhibition of these movements is not possible in all subjects nor for a long time. Szymanski's (1922) subjects, on the command to refrain from movement, performed movements regularly every 0.6-3 min. The findings of Simmons are in agreement with these figures (according to Johnson and Swan, 1930).

A mere glance at the actogram is sufficient to indicate that the hours of waking are, in the majority of cases, clearly distinguishable from the hours of sleep. We have also carried out tests on a number of subjects—we traced the recorded movements after the command: "Lie perfectly still!" and found that even with active inhibition, the majority of them, while awake, could not completely refrain from making small movements, and so failed

40

to present a pattern resembling sleep. We also investigated how long a person could lie motionless in a waking state (without a special task to carry out). In the majority of subjects the intervals of complete rest rarely exceeded 8 min. Only certain individual exceptions (one subject had Parkinsonian akinesia) could lie motionless for longer periods and at the same time react to a signal (see below). In order to establish the fact that definite distinctions could be made between states of sleep and wakefulness on the basis of motor activity, a special investigation was carried out (Andreev, 1951) on another function, connected with the condition of the cerebral cortex—the conditioned reflex activity brought about by a special command, and the trends of both functions were studied during sleep and in the waking state. The conditioned stimulus was the soft sound of a muffled buzzer, and the response reaction—in accordance with the command—light contact of the finger with a rubber bulb in the subject's hand or near it. Signals were investigated the whole night at 1 min intervals, so that periods in which conditioned reflex activity was present could be studied with an accuracy of up to 1 min (Fig. 5). The results obtained in 28 persons (49 investigations in all) showed a parallel relationship between the disappearance of intensive motor activity and the conditioned motor reactions on sleeping and their reappearance on waking.

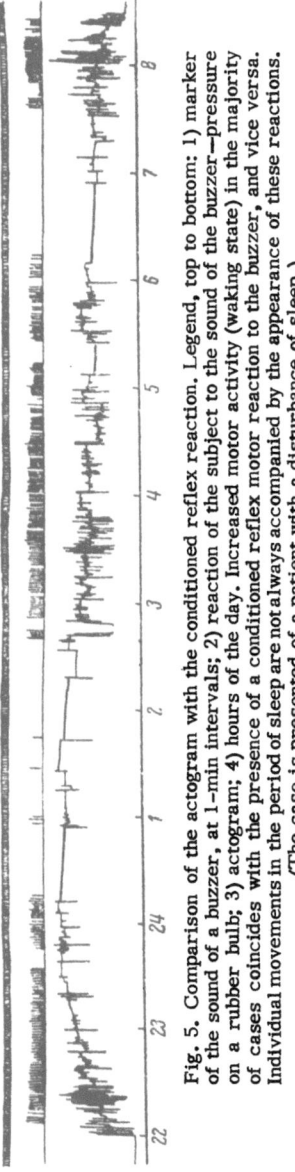

Fig. 5. Comparison of the actogram with the conditioned reflex reaction. Legend, top to bottom: 1) marker of the sound of a buzzer, at 1-min intervals; 2) reaction of the subject to the sound of the buzzer—pressure on a rubber bulb; 3) actogram; 4) hours of the day. Increased motor activity (waking state) in the majority of cases coincides with the presence of a conditioned reflex motor reaction to the buzzer, and vice versa. Individual movements in the period of sleep are not always accompanied by the appearance of these reactions. (The case is presented of a patient with a disturbance of sleep.)

In evaluating the actograms, the verbal account of the subject is always taken into consideration. But these subjective accounts did not always coincide with the data of the actograms. The differences found were usually due to the inaccuracy of the subjective impressions of the patients, which was revealed either by checking on the actual events or by the testimony of third persons.

These findings showed that actography may be used as an objective instrument during sleep and wakefulness in order to solve certain problems, and in particular, during sleep therapy.

SLEEP THERAPY IN THE NEUROSES

CASE MATERIAL

The material for this book is derived from the consideration of a group of 91 patients (Andreev, 1956). The majority were suffering from neuroses: 34 with neurasthenia and 42 with hysteria. The rest of the cases were diagnosed as neurasthenic states caused by somatogenic factors, mild reactive depressions, encephalopathies with neurotic symptomatology, and certain other forms of neurosis. In 19 of the patients with neurasthenia the background was predominantly asthenic, and only in 5 patients was increased excitation observed; the rest showed mixed forms. Most of the patients with hysteria (23) showed asthenic and depressive features, and only 7 patients showed increased excitation, the rest having mixed forms. The syndromes most often seen were phobias and anxiety syndromes (17 patients). A number of the patients had a history of some somatic weakness or disorder such as an endocrine disturbance (hyperthyroidism, menopause) or some previous illness. In a small number of cases the neuroses were complicated by hypertension or peptic ulcers.

METHOD OF TREATMENT

As we have already said above, different methods of sleep therapy are used in the psychoses, and especially in schizophrenia. These methods must be differentiated in accordance with the form and stage of the disease.

In the sleep treatment of neuroses, in which the inhibition is, in the majority of cases, restorative and protective in character, the treatment should consist in the strengthening of this inhibition with a sleep that is as close to physiological as possible, and without any accompanying toxicosis.

In these cases, the protective inhibition was maintained and strengthened by the creation of a favorable environment and by the use of hypnogenic, conditioned reflex factors in the form of direct and verbal stimuli. We used hypnotic drugs in small doses, and in some cases only to create the necessary inhibitory background or to induce conditioned reflex sleep.

An indispensable element in the sleep therapy of neuroses is psychotherapy in the wide sense of the term.

PREPARATION FOR TREATMENT

In the preparatory period, the usual medical examination of the patient was done, the history taken, the patient's personality make-up appraised, the type of his nervous system identified, his higher nervous activity examined by experimental methods, and the diagnosis accurately determined. Before sleep therapy is undertaken it is essential to remove certain obstacles of an interoceptive character, for example by attending to oral hygiene (we have had some cases where toothache has disrupted the course of sleep therapy); other pains of somatic origin must be eliminated, the bowels regularized, cough eradicated, etc.

In sleep therapy it is desirable that the preparatory period be as short as possible—in fact the minimum time necessary to carry out only the most essential tests. The sooner sleep therapy begins, the more effective it will be and the shorter will be the patient's stay in the hospital.

If it is now generally considered to be essential that a psychotherapeutic approach be used (action through the secondary signal system) in any form of treatment, and especially in drug treatment, this is all the more necessary in sleep therapy. We accordingly prepare the patients psychotherapeutically by talking to them. The meaning and nature of the Pavlovian method of sleep therapy is explained to them and they are given instructions on the plan of the treatment to which they must conform. These measures insure the active cooperation of the patients in their treatment. It is also explained to the patients that contact with the outside world during sleep therapy interferes with the success of the treatment.

FORMS OF THERAPEUTIC SLEEP

Various forms of therapeutic sleep are in use. Strel'chuk (1952) lists six forms used in psychoses and neuroses at the clinic of the Institute of Higher Nervous Activity of the Academy of Sciences of the USSR.

We are of the opinion that a classification of the forms of therapeutic sleep in neuroses should be established, based on the daily duration and depth of sleep, the number of interruptions, and the length of the course of treatment. So far as the methods of inducing sleep are concerned, on the basis of which Strel'chuk distinguishes various forms, at the present time nearly all authors, when treating neuroses, try to use functional methods of induction and maintenance of sleep and to reduce as far as possible the use of sedative drugs. In our opinion, two forms of therapeutic sleep are the most suitable for the treatment of neuroses:

1) Interrupted prolonged (fractionated) sleep, closely resembling natural sleep, with two or three interruptions in the 24-hour period.

2) Prolonged nocturnal sleep, used in mild forms of neuroses.

We have used prolonged interrupted, or fractionated sleep, with periods of sleep interrupted by periods of wakefulness three times a day. For our group of patients we favor this form of treatment. The mere prolongation of nocturnal sleep, even if extended to the equivalent daily period of fractionated sleep, cannot make it as valuable as the latter form. Nature itself tells us that, in all cases where the cortex is either not yet fully developed (in babies) or enfeebled by a pathological process (narcolepsy, concussion, infection, etc.), sleep is polyphasic in character, and this consequently is a physiological measure of defense. A reduction in the duration of the period of continuous waking protects the weakened cortex against exhaustion and has a restorative role.

A similar opinion was expressed by Shchelovanov (1954, who considers it most important not simply to prolong sleep, which may not always be possible, but to shorten the periods of waking. He bases his opinion on the ontogenesis of human sleep. In treatment by protective inhibition it is essential to shorten the periods of waking during the day, by interposing one or more periods of sleep. In order to make sleep easier and deeper, Shchelovanov recommends organizing more active employment of the waking periods.

It is difficult to obtain prolonged, continuous sleep without resorting to large doses of sedative drugs. Furthermore, exces-

45

sively prolonged periods of sleep have a number of disadvantages. Movement and some degree of muscular work are physiologically just as necessary to the body as sleep, food, etc. Contractions of the skeletal musculature promote normal blood flow in the veins (Ivanov, 1949, p. 527). Prolonged confinement to bed is known also to interfere with the activity of the gastrointestinal tract (constipation).

Our own personal experience teaches us that too much bed confinement often leads to a feeling of exhaustion of the entire body. Our observations on patients maintained in a state of prolonged induced sleep for several days (for example patient M-va of Dr. M. M. Suslova) also indicate that the patients develop a feeling of exhaustion after this procedure.

In order to compensate for the disadvantages of prolonged recumbency, in a group of patients we prescribed easy gymnastic exercises in bed after waking, under the direction of an instructor, and this made them feel better.

Once a week we interrupted the sleep therapy and prescribed sedation only at night.

PROGRAM FOR THE DAY

The program for the day was built up in accordance with the form of therapeutic sleep used. The morning period of sleep began at 10 a.m. and was allowed to continue until lunch, i.e., until 2 p.m., although the patients usually got up by themselves sooner; the patients went to bed a second time after lunch, at 3 p.m., and were allowed to sleep until supper, i.e., until 7 p.m., but most of them again awoke sooner. They retired for the night's sleep at 10 p.m. In the morning the patients were up from 8 a.m. until 9 a.m.

In the intervals between sleeping, they attended to their toilet, took their meals outside the ward, and could occupy themselves with handwork, light reading, and so on. We tried as far as possible to isolate the patients from the outside world so that no external impressions of an excitatory or disturbing character could interfere with the protective therapy. In any case we did not allow the patients to go outside their own department or to attend meetings of a cultural nature.

Indoor games were also excluded from the patients' routine during the course of sleep therapy. Games such as chess require

46

considerable mental concentration, which is incompatible with the observance of a protective regimen, and if a game is lost, patients often become extremely excited, and it takes a long time before they return to their normal routine. In patient S-v (case No. 794, 1954), who played chess in the intervals between sleep, we observed a deterioration in his sleep and general condition, until the game was prohibited.

On Saturdays the patients took a bath for purposes of hygiene. Since this involved a slight delay in beginning the morning sleep, the patients were not given sedative drugs Saturday mornings, and the duration of the daily sleep was thus slightly shortened.

In cases when we interrupted the sleep therapy and allowed the usual visitors, experience showed that this often upset the patients' equilibrium, disturbed their sleep and, in most cases, made them feel worse. Of course it was occasionally desirable to allow a few patients to have visitors during the course of treatment, but only when such meetings brought an element of tranquillity and not of discord.

More or less similar observations are made by the French authors Sapir and Levy (1953). They consider that the problem of visitors should be solved individually and, in any case, the visitors should first be warned and given suitable instructions, and the time of the interview should not be given precisely, for any accidental delay in the visit would probably nullify the tranquillizing effect of the meeting. Le Guillant (1953) reports that in his clinic visitors are permitted in exceptional cases, but this is always done with care, without the patient's knowledge and without others present in the ward.

THE ENVIRONMENT AND ITS IMPORTANCE

We usually carried out sleep therapy simultaneously on four patients in a ward of four beds, although it might be considered better to have wards of two beds. The administration of sleep therapy on a ward where there were other patients who were not getting sleep treatment proved to be extremely difficult, not very effective and, occasionally even contraindicated. It was regularly found that the fewer patients who shared a room, the less interference there was with sleep. Coughing, snoring, and nocturnal frequency in one of the patients usually meant a loss of rest for the other occupants of the ward. Sleep therapy should not, however, be prescribed for patients in private rooms. Sapir and Levy consider that the treatment of patients in groups stimulates competition, while the necessity for conforming to a common regimen facilitates correct treatment of the group of patients.

We kept the room partially, but not completely, darkened, so that the ward remained dimly lit. This brought the environmental conditions close to those of natural nocturnal sleep. The microclimate—the other environmental conditions—of the ward is of great importance. A temperature above 18-20°C may make it difficult for patients to go to sleep and to sleep soundly. It was shown in Galkin's laboratory (Konstantinov, 1949) that drug-induced sleep is deeper when the environmental temperature is low. In general it would be ideal to carry out sleep therapy in fresh air (on verandas or near open windows), with, of course, suitable furniture and sleeping bags. This method is discussed by Beilin (1951), and others.

The creation of a favorable environment is, of course, of enormous importance for the maintenance of natural physiological sleep. Nowadays, in sleep therapy, it is usual to pay attention to the role of several factors which may produce natural physiological sleep.[1] We consider it desirable to limit these factors to two groups. One comprises everything involved in the protective regimen, and the second consists of stimuli which acquire a conditioned reflex character in this situation. However, frequently they are mixed, and any sleep arising without sedative drugs is called conditioned reflex sleep.

Although the protective regimen is nowadays a component part of almost every form of therapy, in sleep therapy it is an absolutely essential and paramount condition.[2] The complete exclusion of untoward stimuli allows the development of so-called passive sleep. For this purpose the routine of the sleep ward is organized to include insulation from sound, dim lighting, comfortable beds, etc.

---

[1] In reviewing the literature on this subject, we have made use of the experience of authors practicing the sleep treatment of both psychoneuroses and other disorders.

[2] On the importance of the protective regimen, see Beilin, 1951; Chukhrenko, 1952, 1952a; Sizenko, 1952; Obnorskii, 1952; Yurovskii and Maidanskii, 1953.

PHYSICAL HYPNOGENIC FACTORS

To facilitate the development of sleep, in some cases hypnogenic agents are used, in the form of weak, monotonous stimuli.

Some time ago the Pavlov school found that uniform and protracted stimuli, causing fatigue of nerve cells, lead to inhibition in the corresponding area of the cerebral cortex whence it may irradiate to neighboring areas, and often end in sleep.

On the basis of this finding, many authors use various stimuli to produce sleep, for example sound stimuli (a buzzer or metronome, the sound of rain or running water, etc.), light stimuli (a winking green "glowworm"), temperature stimuli (hot water bottle); electrically induced sleep is also largely explained by the action of a weak, rhythmic stimulus. All these are fundamentally unconditioned sleep-producing factors, and it is only after a series of combinations that they acquire the additional property of conditioned stimuli.

Some interesting observations have been made on the action of the various hypnogenic stimuli. Bogachenko (1952), for example, found that a metronome and a winking light with a frequency of 30–60 interruptions per minute prevented children from going to sleep, whereas if the frequency was 15–20 interruptions per minute, it helped them to go to sleep. Ivanov would not use a metronome, for this did not induce sleep, but caused excitation. Ivanov, in contrast to other authors, also considers that hot water bottles make sleep more difficult. The use of hot water bottles evidently calls for an individual approach and no general recommendation can be given. They may help, for instance, in cases when coldness of the limbs prevents the patient from going to sleep.

Aleksandrova and Prokhorova note that the attitude towards a hypnogenic stimulus is an individual one: some patients sleep best in complete silence.

We tested the action of uniform sound stimuli as sleep-producing factors. By analogy with the soporific action of the rhythmic sounds on a steamship or train, we considered that the distant, soft, uniform sound of the motor of our ventilator would tranquillize patients and help them to sleep. In practice, however, our expectations were not borne out. We hardly saw a single case in which the sound of the motor had a beneficial action; some reacted indifferently to it, and others begged to be rid of the noise, for it irritated them and prevented them from sleeping. In one patient this attitude to the stimulus was probably connected with his job. In three patients the negative reaction to the sound of the motor was selective, for another sound (a fountain) had a positive action on them, and only one patient could not tolerate either one. It must be pointed out that not only our motor, but also the weak sounds from other motors, sometimes carried up from the lower floors of the building, or through the open windows from the street, or from nearby factories, also affected the patients unfavorably and disturbed their sleep, though they would not be noticed by healthy persons.

We once tried to use a metronome as a hypnogenic stimulus, but then had to give it up for the following reason: even when it was put in a box to deaden the sound, in the majority of cases it did not tranquillize nor induce drowsiness, but, on the contrary, irritated the patients, and they asked for its removal. In many cases this negative attitude towards the metronome in Leningrad citizens was connected with the blockade period, when the sound of a metronome was heard from loudspeakers in the intervals between radio transmissions and throughout the night.

One of the uniform sound stimuli which encouraged sleep was a small fountain, consisting of thin jets of water. It gives a soft sound, slightly reminiscent of the sound of rain. Almost all patients (we used it in sleep therapy in 35 patients) reacted favorably to this stimulus, declaring that it had a pleasant effect, was soothing, and assisted sleep. Only the one patient mentioned above, who was suffering from hysteria, could tolerate neither the sound of the fountain nor the other sounds. In some cases the fountain was not turned on during the first day of the course of treatment, and then patients who knew its purpose themselves asked for it to be set in motion. We had such a request from seven patients. Four of these later explained that absolute quiet is depressing: "Thoughts fly through your head, and the sound of the fountain helps you to go to sleep."

Of course, neither the fountain alone, nor any other monotonous stimulus, can be considered sufficient to induce sleep at any particular time. In the same way, a sedative drug alone, when given in ordinary doses, does not always induce sleep unless all the necessary conditions are observed. The monotonous sound of dripping water, if used together with other factors, and especially in combination with very small doses of sedatives, undoubtedly helps to induce and maintain sleep, for, by imitating rain, it is a stimulus which in natural conditions promotes sound sleep.

THE USE OF SEDATIVES

In the treatment of neuroses, many physicians were unwilling to give large doses of sedatives, since they did not produce sound sleep but, on the contrary, often led to signs of excitation and to toxic effects (Zaretskii, Ivanov, Yakovleva, 1952). A tendency is generally observed for the total amount of sedative drugs administered during the course of treatment to be reduced; many use conditioned reflex sleep, produced in response to inert substitutes for sedatives ("conditioned sedatives") and a combination of soporific stimuli from the environment as a whole. Some physicians try to carry out sleep therapy by the use of hypnosis and suggestion alone (see below).

As sedative agents we have usually used the barbiturates: phenobarbital, usually in doses of 0.05−0.1 g each; sodium amytal, 0.1−0.2 g; less often nembutal, 0.1 g; veronal, 0.2−0.3 g; and medinal in the same dose. By using small doses, and without bringing patients to the point of toxic manifestations, we were unable to detect any significant difference between the actions of these various sedatives and to preferentially select one of them. In some cases the barbiturate was supplemented with chloral hydrate in doses of 0.6−1.6 g. Sometimes it helped very little, but in a few cases it was only this combination that produced an effect.

Individual partiality for a particular sedative, when the patient tolerates one drug badly and others well, may be explained in some cases by conditioned reflex mechanisms and not by an unconditioned action. If on one occasion the patient is not feeling well while taking a particular drug, this may reinforce this connection through a conditioned reflex mechanism, and the patient may subsequently show intolerance to this drug and complete tolerance to another which closely resembles it in nature. We were convinced of the conditioned origin of such an "idiosyncrasy" in two patients. Patient Kh-n, suffering from hysteria, was given an inert powder, one night, that was supposed to be a sedative. The patient, convinced that she had been given phenobarbital, which had previously made her feel ill, complained next morning of giddiness and nausea and of having spent a bad night. In patient M-i we observed another variant of this conditioned reflex effect. This patient was also prejudiced against phenobarbital which, in her own words, she tolerated badly, and she preferred medinal. When, however, she was given phenobarbital disguised as medinal, she slept well and experienced no unpleasant sensations.

With regard to dosage, we were guided by this principle: never to bring patients to the stage where they show toxic manifestations. Every day, on morning rounds, and also during the daytime interval, we asked the patients how they felt and observed their condition, and if mention was made of unpleasant sensations or symptoms, the next dose of the drug was either withheld, or we substituted a "conditioned powder," or reduced the dose. The patients were thus kept in good spirits and feeling well throughout treatment; in their outward appearance and behavior they were completely indistinguishable from the rest of the patients.

We avoided giving combinations of sedatives (except for chloral hydrate with barbiturates in a few cases) for the following reasons: in order to elucidate certain problems of treatment methods, it was necessary to vary the dose of one hypnotic only. If we had used combinations of drugs, it would have made analysis of the action more difficult.

In their practice of sleep therapy, many workers employ different combinations. A series of mixtures is available, each named after their authors (Asratyan, Grashchenkov, Ivanov-Smolenskii). We have not, however, found any clinical observations which convincingly proved that one mixture is better than another, or that a mixture is better than one drug alone. On the other hand, experimental work on animals shows that if a given combination has a potentiating action on animals of one species, quite different results may be obtained on animals of a closely related species (Hesse, Baumgart, and Dickmann, 1932, and others). Care must be taken, however, in applying to man experimental data obtained from animals. The question of the superiority of certain combinations of hypnotics after experimental investigations on animals calls for special study in man.

In general, Pavlov[1] was against giving complicated mixtures containing a large number of ingredients for the same reason, namely, the impossibility of understanding the mechanism of action of the drugs used. Later on, Pavlov recognized that it was worth while giving a combination of bromide and caffeine, but only after a careful study of the mechanism of action of each component separately and a prolonged experimental trial of this combination. Le Guillant later declared against the use of various mixtures (cocktails, as he called them) in sleep therapy.

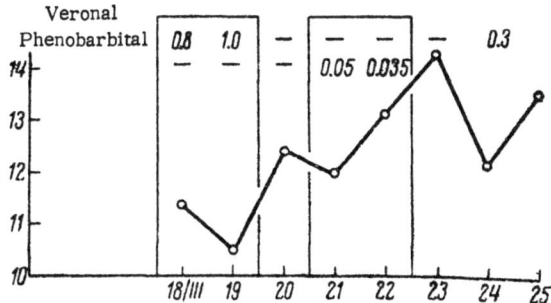

Fig. 6. Pattern of daily duration of sleep in patient Sm–a after varying dosage of sedatives. Along the horizontal axis the day of the month is indicated, and along the vertical axis, the number of hours of sleep within 24 hours. The figures above the points on the curve indicate the daily dose of the sedative named on the left. Average doses of sedative (veronal) shorten the duration of sleep (March 18, 19, and 24). On the evening of the 18th unmotivated tears were observed in this patient. On the 19th, a state of excitation was observed, with tears after administration of 0.5 g veronal in the morning and afternoon. The best effects were obtained by the action of the residual doses of the sedatives (on the next day: March 20, 23, and 25).

So far as the use of the popular combinations of sedatives (barbiturates) with bromide is concerned, we have tested these in only a few cases, and generally speaking, have avoided them for the following reason: we know from the work of Petrova (1935), Birman, and Zigel' (1934), and Birman and Vainberg (1935), that optimal doses of bromide concentrate the process of inhibition, dispel drowsiness during the daytime and improve sleep at night, whereas we were trying to produce sleep during

[1] Pavlov's Wednesdays, Vol. 2, p. 298 [in Russian].

the daytime as well, i.e., to produce irradiation of the inhibition. These two drugs, acting antagonistically in these conditions, thus diminish the total effect on day-time sleep. Synergism might, perhaps, be exhibited by these two drugs if the bromide were given in doses exceeding the optimal value.

We were satisfied that in many cases in which bromide was added to a barbiturate, no intensification of the effect nor any reduction of sleep was observed, and only in 2 cases was its use followed by an increase in the duration of sleep in the 24 hours. It is evident that the effect of this combination, whatever it may be, depends on the particular type of patient concerned, and on his condition, so that its use should be determined on a strictly individual basis. In one of our patients the inhibitory symptoms were markedly benefited, and accordingly in this case the use of bromide in the course of sleep therapy played a positive role.

When dosage was fixed, consideration was given to the type of nervous system, although in practice this is a more complicated question than is generally realized. In the first place the degree of strength of the nervous system cannot always be determined

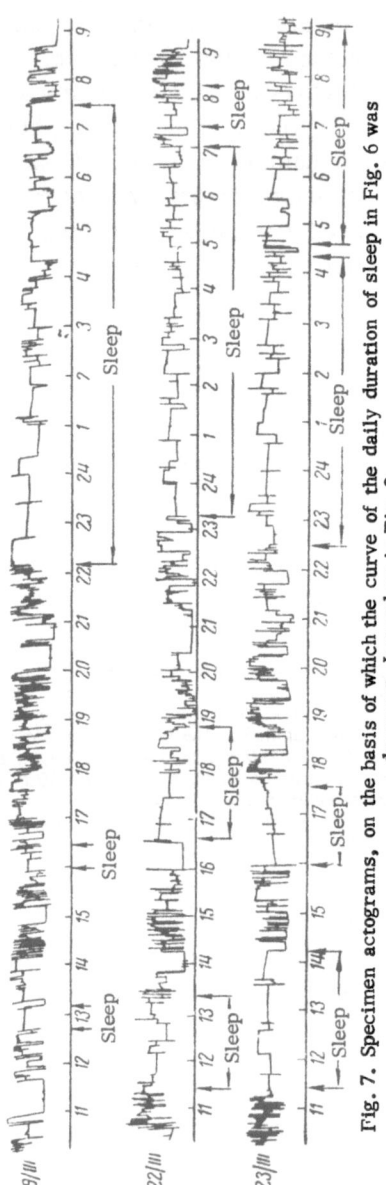

Fig. 7. Specimen actograms, on the basis of which the curve of the daily duration of sleep in Fig. 6 was drawn up. Legend as in Fig. 3.

with sufficient accuracy, and furthermore, the usual strength of the patient's nervous system may be weakened to a varying degree at the time of an illness. Also, it can hardly be asserted categorically that the type as determined on the basis of a person's behavior will be absolutely identical with the "pharmacological" type, i.e., with that determined on the basis of tolerance to a particular drug. This is a matter for further investigation and trial. In the meantime we have been able to obtain only an approximate idea of the type of nervous system and, in the majority of cases, we have first had to test the patient's tolerance to the sedative, starting with small doses. On the other hand, we did not undertake the investigation of the relationship between type and dosage as a special task. We did not always, therefore, push forward to maximal dosage of the sedative used, i.e., the dose was not carried far enough for toxic manifestations to appear,

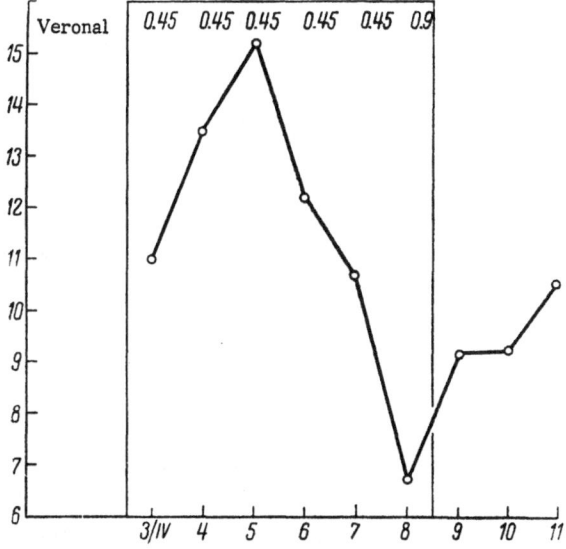

Fig. 8. Pattern of the daily duration of sleep in S-va. Legend as in Fig. 6. Good results in the form of prolonged sleep were produced by small doses of veronal, viz., 0.15 g three times a day. Subsequently the curve for length of sleep began to fall, presumably on account of cumulation of the sedative. Administration of a larger dose of 0.3 g on April 8, to clarify the cause of the fall of the curve, caused toxic manifestations and a sharp fall in the duration of sleep. The inadequate increase in the length of sleep on April 9 and 10 is accounted for by incidental disturbances during the night.

but if the patient slept well after a small test dose, this dose was then maintained without change.

In a group of cases with a weak or weakened nervous system we observed a paradoxical effect after increasing the dose of sedative, i.e., a diminution instead of a prolongation of the period of sleep. In the patient Sm-a (case No. 56, 1950) average doses of veronal shortened the duration of sleep and evoked a reaction in the form of unmotivated crying; the best effect was obtained by the action of the doses of sedatives used thereafter (on the following day; Figs. 6, 7). In the patient S-va (case No. 173, 1950) sound sleep was obtained by the use of small doses of veronal, and an increase in the dose to a moderate value led to a marked reduction of sleep (Figs. 8 and 9). In patient B-ich (case No. 824, 1950) administration of sodium amytal with chloral hydrate at first induced euphoria and a state of excitation; with an increase in the dose of sodium amytal to 1.1 g daily, on the second day the state of excitation was aggravated, the duration of sleep reduced, and the patient began to express suicidal ideas. When sedation was interrupted insomnia developed on the first night, but this was gradually corrected by

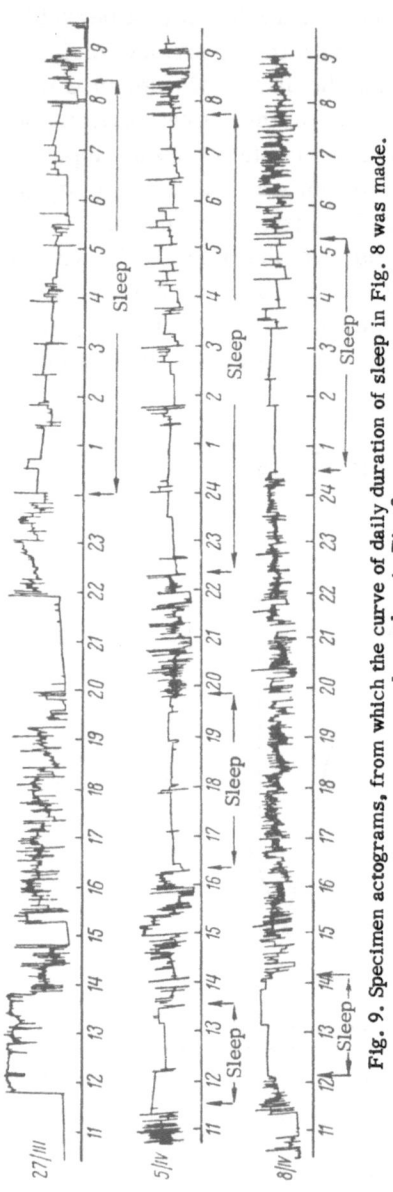

Fig. 9. Specimen actograms, from which the curve of daily duration of sleep in Fig. 8 was made. Legend as in Fig. 3.

the administration of bromural and small doses of other sedatives.

Some authors account for these phenomena by the presence of a paradoxical phase, during which a strong stimulus (a large dose of sedative) elicits a smaller response than a weak stimulus (a small dose). De Guillant regards the development of insomnia or the appearance of excitation under the influence of a sedative as evidence of an ultraparadoxical phase. In these cases, according to his observations, total withdrawal of the hypnotic may abolish the insomnia.

In a group of patients with a strong type of nervous system, the administration of moderate doses of sedatives produced no toxic manifestations. Patient L-va, for instance, received a daily dose of 0.7 g sodium amytal for 15 days with a break on the rest days, and no toxic signs whatever were observed. Patient L-na received a daily dose of 0.45 g nembutal for several days, also with no toxic signs of any sort. In order to ensure better absorption of the sedative and the onset of its action by bedtime, the patients took the drug in the morning and afternoon before meals.

Sedatives were always taken in the presence of the nurse on duty. The patients knew that they were being given a sedative, but neither the name of the drug nor the dose was communicated to them. When the patient is aware of the nature of the powder or capsule which he takes, then with a drop in the dose or substitution of a placebo, the conditioned reflex effect either does not develop or is reduced.

THE USE OF INERT SUBSTANCES (SEDATIVE SUBSTITUTES) AS CONDITIONED REFLEX STIMULI

Nearly all papers on the subject of therapeutic sleep appearing nowadays mention the use of conditioned reflex sleep (Rakhlin, 1948; Beilin, 1951; Lizunova, 1950; Baltsvinik, 1951; Nikulin, 1951; Kamyanov, 1952; Syasev, 1952; Bogachenko, 1952; Kurilenko, 1952; Shpak, 1953; Aleksandrova and Prokhorova, 1953; Shoshin, 1954; Gorodetskaya, 1954). However, the majority of these authors did not do any objective recording of the daily proportion of sleep and wakefulness; in this area the observations of assistants may not be sufficiently complete. In most of these articles no analysis is made of the data on conditioned reflex sleep during the course of treatment.

The authors either give the average number of days necessary for the development of conditioned reflex sleep, or they indicate the point in treatment when the sedatives began to be replaced by placeboes. This varied in different investigations from 3 to 10 days after medication was begun. The conditioned reflex effect lasted from 1 to 6 days, and only Bogachenko asserts that in children it may extend for 21 days after the use of small doses of hypnotics (bromural, 0.05 g). It is difficult to regard a conditioned effect of this duration purely as the result of placebo substitution (glucose), and not as the result of the action of the external environment as a whole, especially since the author himself shows a diagram of the increased duration of sleep in one child who received neither sedatives nor placeboes.

Some workers prescribed sedatives and placeboes in capsule form, but in view of the fact that from time to time patients would chew the capsules, it became necessary to imitate the taste of the sedatives. Kamyanov replaced barbiturates by inert powders with the addition of quinine, and chloral hydrate with the addition of sodium chloride solution. In order to enhance the conditioned reflex effect, Shoshin added peppermint water or anise water to sedatives and placeboes, and Shpak added nicotinic acid. Syasev included a buzzer or a colored lamp to act on other receptors.

The prolongation of sleep obtained by certain workers after replacement of sedatives with other substances was possibly the result not of a conditioned effect, but of residual doses of hypnotics given in large quantities. Syasev, for instance, gave phenobarbital in a daily dose of 0.6 g and chloral hydrate as an enema containing 1.5 g, and under these circumstances observed the development of toxic effects in certain cases. Shpak gave 0.4 g sodium amytal in the morning, 0.2 g phenobarbital in the afternoon and 0.5 g veronal in the evening (obviously a large daily dose).

Nikulin offers a more critical evaluation of the effect of placeboes in his investigations of conditioned reflex sleep. Research in his clinic showed that when the higher nervous activity is of the excited type, usually no conditioned reflex effect is obtained from the administration of inert substances, and if an effect is obtained, it quickly becomes extinguished. A paradoxical effect often arises, i.e., instead of sleep, excitation is induced. When the higher nervous activity is of an inhibited nature, the duration of conditioned reflex sleep is considerable and it may last for several days. The author presents a curve showing that on the day of replacement of the sedative by the conditioned powders, the duration of sleep even increased, but he does not show the initial basal duration of sleep and he does not state what doses of sedative were used (for reinforcement).

There remains the possibility that this conditioned effect is due to the action of a residual level of sedative remaining in the body on the following day representing at this time an optimal dose compared with the usual massive dose.

Kurilenko points out that no conditioned reflex sleep is produced in excited patients. In attempting to induce conditioned reflex sleep, Gorodetskaya used placeboes 4–5 days after sound sleep had been induced by sedatives, and states that as a rule he was unable to obtain conditioned reflex sleep for more than 24 hours at a time. Often such sleep was maintained only after the next one or two doses of the placebo. Simonov (1954) describes the results of clinical observations which are in agreement with our own. He writes that he repeatedly had to contend with a sharp reduction of sleep in patients who received placeboes for a long time without reinforcement with sedatives. When the patient again received the same dose of sedative (or even a slightly larger dose), as a rule for two or three nights he did not sleep as well as he did before he was given the placeboes. This phenomenon is explained by irradiation of the active inhibition (during extinction) which also affects the unconditioned reaction. On the third and fourth night sleep was restored with the same dose of sedative.

The search for methods of treatment by means of protective inhibition without toxic manifestations led us to conduct a special investigation on the use of conditioned reflex sleep, in which sedatives were replaced by inert substances. As a substitute we used sugar, to which quinine was added in order to give it a bitter taste similar to the sedatives, and sugar was also added to small doses of the sedative. The weight of the powder, regardless of the dose or material involved, was 0.5 g, i.e., it was almost the same in each case.

The patients subsequently received sedatives and their inert substitutes in gelatin capsules which, it was thought, would prevent them from distinguishing the taste of the drug given. Some patients, however, chewed the capsule, so that we had to continue imitating the taste, and we thought it desirable to use semolina as the substitute, as recommended by certain authors. The question still remains, however, whether by using capsules we are not depriving ourselves of an additional and quite powerful component of the conditioned stimulus in the form of the sensation of taste. When preparing to dispense the medicines, the nurse wrote on the wrapper of the powder only the patient's surname and, as we have already stated, the patient did not know what sedative he was taking.

Investigation in human subjects of the conditioned pharmacological effect, as indicated by the onset of sleep, in the course of sleep therapy is an extremely complicated and time-consuming task. In the first place, reliable results can only be obtained when the duration of sleep during the course of treatment differs considerably from the initial basal level, and this is not invariably the case. If the difference does not exceed 2 hours, let us say, variations from incidental causes may be found within the same limits, and the results obtained would not provide a sufficient basis for conclusions. Furthermore, the presence or absence of a conditioned reflex effect can be clearly noted only if great variations in the duration of sleep are not observed from day to day, in response to various accidental factors. One, two or three tests may be performed on each patient, for in the event of a negative effect, the action of the unconditioned stimulus—the sedative—is also inhibited on the following day. When the course of treatment lasts two or three weeks, with breaks on Sundays, the number of tests may thus be very limited. In view of these considerations, we carried out investigations on patients who satisfied the above-mentioned conditions.

In a group of 26 patients with various neuroses, we attempted to produce conditioned reflex sleep following the use of phenobarbital in daily doses of 0.1 to 0.3 g. The tests were performed at different times, starting on the second day after administration of sedatives and ending on the 22nd day. One test was made and, if a conditioned effect was obtained, occasionally we carried out a series of several tests in order to investigate the duration of extinction of the conditioned effect.

In five patients no conditioned effect was obtained, although in two of them the test was performed twice (in one on the 4th and 12th day of administration of the sedative and in the other on the 9th and 15th day). In four patients the effect was doubtful, i.e., on the day the placebo was given the duration of sleep was considerably shortened, but not to its initial level. In 17 patients

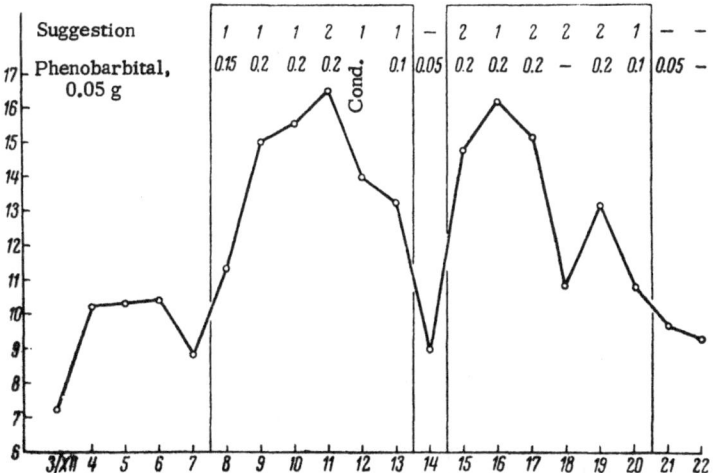

Fig. 10. Pattern of the daily duration of sleep. Legend as in Fig. 6. The top row of figures indicates the number of sessions of suggestion during the given day. The points on the curve which are not included inside the rectangles correspond to days on which sleep therapy was interrupted. The remark "Cond." indicates the administration of conditioned powders. Withdrawal of sedative, while maintaining all the other conditions, on December 18 evokes a sharp decrease in the duration of sleep. On December 12, when the sedative is replaced by the placebo, conditioned reflex sleep is observed.

a positive conditioned effect was obtained. In order to differentiate between the conditioned effect resulting from administration of the inert powder and the conditioned effect from the environment as a whole, as well as the effect of residual traces of sedative, in some patients on certain days we gave neither sedatives nor placeboes; in these cases a sharp fall in the duration of sleep was observed (Figs. 10 and 11). In other, and evidently rarer cases, both the sedative itself and its substitute play a secondary role, and the prolongation of sleep is brought about by a pre-existing marked tendency toward protective inhibition and by the influence of the environment as a whole, promoting the development of sleep.

When conditioned powders were given repeatedly for several successive days, we observed extinction of the conditioned effect. Seventeen tests were carried out in succession on 11 patients, with other factors unchanged. Usually on the second or third day

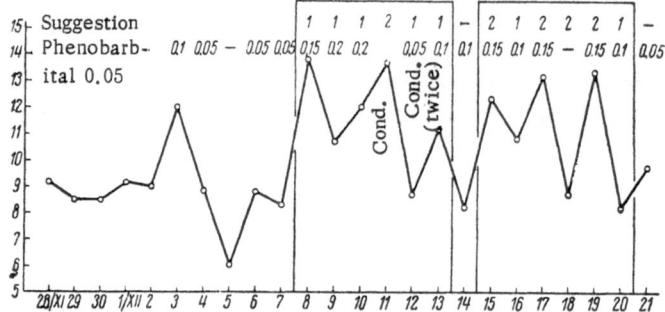

Fig. 11. Pattern of the daily duration of sleep. Legend as in Fig. 10. Extinction of the conditioned effect on the second day (December 12) after administration of the placebo, in spite of reinforcement with a very small dose of sedative; duration of sleep the same as without sedative and placebo (test on December 18).

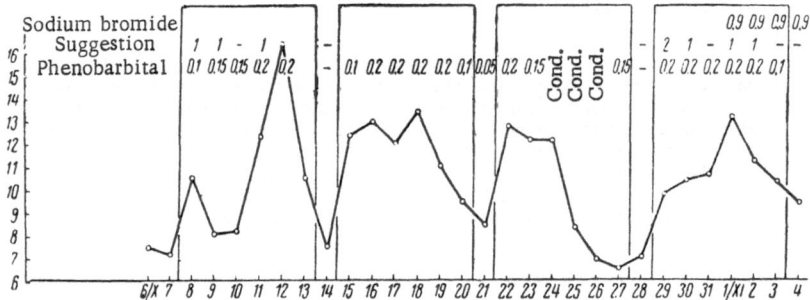

Fig. 12. Pattern of the daily duration of sleep. Legend as in Fig. 10. Extinction of the conditioned reflex effect after the second administration of the placebo (October 25). Administration of placebo as a control test for a third trial caused an even greater fall in the curve of duration of sleep. Next day, in spite of reinforcement with sedation, inhibition of the unconditioned reaction is observed. The curve later returns only gradually to the previous level.

the duration of sleep was reduced to its original level (Figs. 12, 13, and 14). We avoided frequent repetition of test periods with placeboes, especially those lasting three days, for in cases where the results were negative the resulting loss of sleep had an adverse effect on the condition of the patients, and sedatives given on the days immediately after extinction were less effective (Figs. 12 and 13).

The cause of failure in a certain number of cases might have been the use of small doses of sedatives, which made the formation of the conditioned connection more difficult.

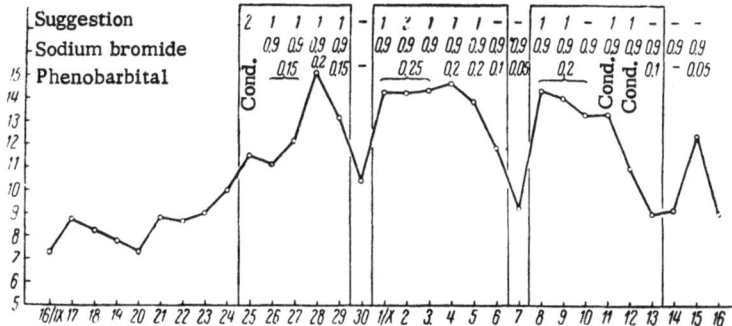

Fig. 13. Pattern of the daily duration of sleep. Legend as in Fig. 10. By the use of placeboes on two consecutive days (October 11 and 12), extinction of the effect developed on the second day. Next day, in spite of reinforcement with sedation, the curve of duration of sleep fell even lower: inhibition of the unconditioned effect took place.

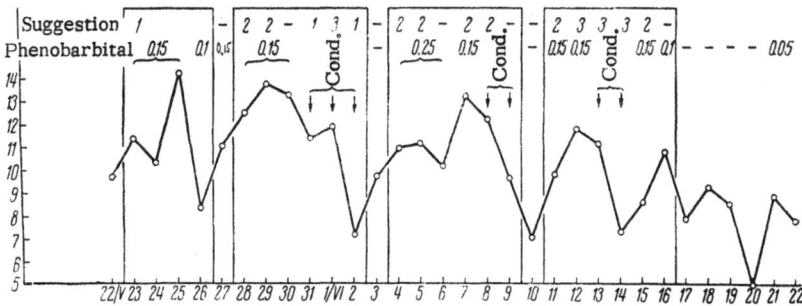

Fig. 14. Pattern of the daily duration of sleep. Legend as in Fig. 10. When placeboes are used for several days in succession, in the first trial (May 31—June 2) extinction of the conditioned reflex effect appears on the third day, and in the second trial (June 8—9) the effect is doubtful on the second day. The insufficient length of sleep on June 20 is due to other causes.

In five cases, during a course of treatment with sodium amytal in daily doses of 0.2 to 0.7 g, when this was replaced by placeboes no effect could be obtained, in spite of the fact that in one patient the test was carried out on the 24th day of administration of sedatives, in another on the 16th and 17th day, and in a third on the 5th, 10th, and 15th days. We think that this failure with sodium amytal is due to its specific taste, which cannot be reproduced by means of an assortment of inert mixtures; in these circumstances the patients often knew that they were being given another sedative.

Our investigation on conditioned reflex sleep thus showed that it must be used carefully, avoiding prolonged (for several successive days) replacement of sedatives by inert substances, in order to prevent the development of persistent extinction of the conditioned effect, followed by irradiation of the inhibition, depriving the sedatives of their unconditioned action. Careful watch must be kept for the presence of the conditioned reflex effect, and it must frequently be reinforced by the addition of small doses of sedatives.

So far as the connection between the mechanism of the conditioned reflex effect and the form of the disease or type of nervous system is concerned, the material that we have accumulated does not yet permit definite conclusions. There is an apparent tendency, however, toward the greater ease of formation of a conditioned effect in persons of artistic type. Of the 15 patients in whom such an effect was produced, 9 were of the artistic type. In the group of 9 persons in whom the result was negative, there was only one patient of artistic type, though a very excitable case. [According to Pavlov the "artistic" type is characterized by the relative prominence of the primary, as compared with the secondary, signal system—Editor.]

THE USE OF HYPNOSIS AND SUGGESTION

Sleep treatment induced by hypnosis without the use of any form of sedative drug can be regarded as ideal in neurotic states of various kinds. Hypnosis has been used for a long time in therapeutic practice in two directions: as "hypnosis—relaxation," i.e., prolonged sleep, and as a condition in which the patient is more susceptible to suggestion, so that various therapeutic suggestions can become effective. Although the second is popular enough, the first was less so until recently. Nevertheless even the old hypnotists—Liebeault (1866), Beaunis (1899), Wetterstrand (1891), Grasset (1903), Vogt (1895), etc.—used this method of treatment and recommended it.

Petrova, of the Pavlov school, working with dogs, showed by numerous experiments the remedial protective effect of hypnotic sleep on the recovery from experimentally induced disturbances of conditioned reflex activity, the abolition of "depth phobias", and even on the disappearance of certain vegetative-trophic disorders. For the treatment of dogs in a state of decrepitude, and also of dogs suffering from chronic neuroses, Petrova (1946) in some cases used veronal sleep and in others hypnotic, i.e., sleep induced by physiological means (by monotonous stimuli and conditioned inhibitory agents). This author thought very highly of hypnotic sleep; because of its special action, more pronounced and more persistent results were obtained than by pharmacological sleep. The deeper the hypnotic sleep, the more quickly did recovery of the disturbed nervous equilibrium of the animal take place, and the dystrophic changes in the skin disappear.

Platonov (1952) repeatedly drew attention to the importance of this therapeutic procedure. Hypnotic sleep, when applied to man, inevitably includes elements of suggestion and autosuggestion, which increases its therapeutic value still more. This author carried out an experimental investigation in the laboratory, which showed that the restoration of working capacity and the increase in pulmonary ventilation after work on an ergograph during even transient hypnotic sleep take place more quickly than when awake. An improvement in the working capacity of the cortical cells after hypnotic sleep was observed by Suslova (1956).

Rozhnov (1953) used therapeutic suggestion in a group of patients with mainly neurotic conditions, and was convinced that in cases when a hypnotic seance of short duration did not help, its therapeutic value was tremendously increased after longer (1–1½ hours) sessions, i.e., when suggestion was combined with hypnotic sleep.

From the foregoing, it thus appears that hypnotic sleep is one of the most valuable forms of remedial protective inhibition. At the same time, there are limitations to the use of hypnotic sleep, for its induction depends on the degree of hypnosuggestibility of the patient. Hypnotists in former days could not explain the factors with which hypnosuggestibility is connected or on which it depends. It was merely known to be absent in young children and in many psychotic states, and diminished in old age. With regard to other conditions, only a small number of observations were made. Many authors pointed out that it was more difficult to induce suggestion and hypnosis in persons with leanings toward reasonableness, analytic tendencies, extreme introspection, critical and skeptical traits. (Bekhterev, 1900; Moll, 1924; Forel, 1928; Löwenfeld, 1928; and others). It was also observed that the functional state plays an important role here: physical and mental exhaustion facilitate induction of hypnosis, and it was therefore recommended that hypnosis be induced after dinner or in the evening, etc.

It was only as a result of Pavlov's study of the physiological mechanisms of hypnosis and suggestion that it became possible to establish the connection between hypnosuggestibility, the type of the nervous system and the form of the neurosis. This problem was further considered by Birman (1934). He considered that at the two opposite poles of degree of hypnosuggestibility are to be found persons in which there is dominance of one of the two signal systems, and a background of predominant excitation or inhibition. For instance, group 1 neuroses (an extreme group with absence of hypnosuggestibility) include forms of irritative neurasthenia and psychasthenia with obsessions; group 2 (by degree of hypnosuggestibility)—less pronounced forms of irritative neurasthenia and psychasthenia; group 3 (more readily hypnotized) includes forms of neurasthenia of a depressive type, reactive depressions, anxiety neuroses and hystero-neurasthenia;[1] group 4 (suggestion rapidly induced, with marked susceptibility to hypnosis)—hysteria of infantile type; and group 5 (suggestion rapidly induced, deep phases of hypnosis) includes constitutional forms of hysteria.[2] Thus, when equilibrium is disturbed towards predominance of the secondary signal system and the process of excitation is pronounced, the hypnosuggestibility is diminished, and conversely, when the secondary signal system is weak and

[1]This term is hardly ever used nowadays in the formulation of the diagnosis.

[2] Birman understood by the word "constitutional" a disease, developing and becoming firmly established in the course of life, in contrast to "reactive", in which an accidental episode arises under the influence of acute psychogenic factors.

the tonus of the cortex is decreased, the hypnosuggestibility is increased.

Strel'chuk (1955), on the basis of modern ideas, carried out investigations of the methods of application of hypnosis, depending on the relationship between the signal systems. In hysteria, for example, it is easier to induce a state of hypnosis by verbal suggestion. This procedure creates an isolated focus of excitation, but the secondary signal system, being weakened, cannot function as a whole and resists the cogency of the suggestion. In psychasthenia, verbal suggestion has a weak action, for the focus of excitation arising here is always under the control of the relatively strong secondary signal system. In this case the patient is more easily put into a hypnotic state by direct monotonous stimuli, the soporific action of which is exerted through the enfeebled primary signal system. Guided by these concepts, we can give a tentative answer to the question of the limitations of hypnosis and of its mode of action in a given patient.

Several authors have described the use of therapeutic sleep, employing suggestion during hypnosis alone (without sedative drugs) in groups of patients (Bunin and Sinitsin, 1951; Levina and Terletskaya, 1951; Rashkovan, 1951; Druzhinin, 1953). Rashkovan sometimes carried out suggestion over the telephone or transferred the rapport to the nurse in charge.

We did not have a large enough number of patients in whom hypnosis was easily induced for therapeutic sleep to be maintained by means of suggestion alone. There is no doubt that the use of hypnotic sleep alone is at present insufficient for treatment by protective inhibition; it is equally clear that it cannot be considered in all cases and that it cannot dispense completely with sedative drugs. In cases in which the ability to undergo hypnosis is diminished, the use of a small dose of some sedative is recommended before the hypnotic session, in order to create a favorable inhibitory background (Löwenthal, Moll, Strel'chuk, Platonov, and many others).

Ivanov-Smolenskii (1951) and Strel'chuk (1952) recommended prolonged hypnotic sleep lasting 18–22 hours for several days in succession in neurotic states and addictions (assumedly in those cases where the susceptibility to hypnosis is sufficiently marked).

When giving sleep therapy, we used hypnotic suggestion as one of the conditioned reflex factors. Usually, after the onset of hypnotic sleep, a combination was used of the method of kinesthetic stimuli (as described by Birman, 1934) — ocular convergence by focusing the eyes on the index finger, with the verbal suggestion of sleep. Later, by means of various tests, we determined the presence of a particular stage of hypnosis.

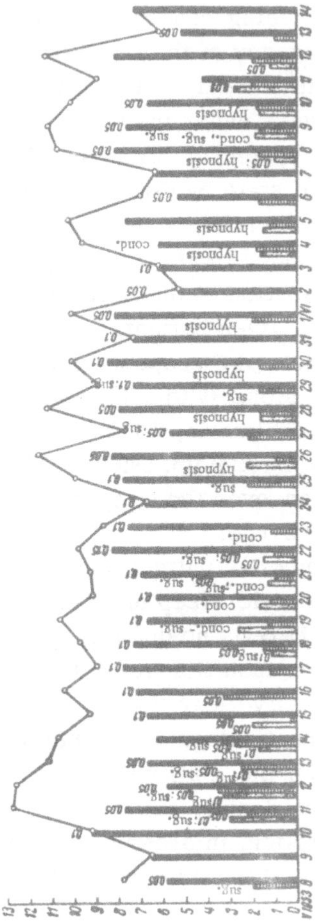

In some cases we carried out hypnosis in a separate room, and then took the patient back to the ward to sleep. In other cases we induced hypnotic sleep in the patient in his bed, and afterwards he was left there to continue his sleep.

It is clear from Fig. 15 that on days of hypnosis, when patient M-va (case No. 330, 1953) had sleep induced by suggestion, usually in the morning, the curve of the daily duration of sleep rose appreciably (May 26, 28, and 30 and June 1, 4, 5, 8, and 10).

In cases when we confined ourselves to a brief 3 to 5 min period of suggestion of sleep in the ward, without awaiting the onset of a deeper stage of hypnosis, the observed effect was less pronounced, i.e., the sleep on

Fig. 15. The effect of hypnosis and sedative drugs on the duration of sleep in M-va. Legend as in Fig. 6. Top—curve of the daily duration of sleep. The columns indicate the duration of sleep in hours: stippled— morning sleep, hatched—afternoon sleep, and black—night sleep. Marks opposite the columns: doses of phenobarbital, "sug." means suggestion, "cond." means conditioned (inert) powders. The inadequate length of sleep on May 9 and 30 (morning) and June 11 was due to other causes.

May 19 (placeboes and suggestion in the morning and afternoon); on May 20 only placeboes were given.

The second cycle of treatment generally resulted in slightly increased figures for the hours of sleep, in spite of the smaller dose of sedative drugs given, which was associated with the more relaxed condition of the patient; also, some of the external obstacles to sleep, previously present, had been removed.

Induction of a state of hypnosis in order to bring about immediate prolongation of sleep was successful in a group of patients, but only in the absence of obstacles and by the observance of other necessary conditions. When, for some reason or other, it was impossible to carry out a long session of hypnosis, we used sleep by brief suggestion. The physician visited each patient preparing to go to sleep and, for a period of 3 to 5 minutes, uttered a predetermined formula, slightly modified for individual circumstances, evoking ideas of rest and sleep.

It was shown both by the expressions of the patients and by objective recording and analysis that this brief suggestion had a beneficial action by facilitating the onset of sleep. All the patients reacted favorably to the suggestion of sleep, declaring that it soothed them and helped them to sleep more quickly. From the actograms we examined in a small number of patients, involving cases in which sleep took place with and without the use of suggestion, we were satisfied that suggestion undoubtedly promotes sleep (see Table 1). In response to suggestion, patients K-va and Gr-r usually slept within 20 minutes, but without suggestion these patients were not asleep, in the majority of cases, in that period of time.

In the absence of the physician in the evening, in some cases the suggestion used was recorded on a tape and played back by the duty nurse. Although the presence of the physician is one of the main factors determining the effectiveness of psychotherapy, and of hypnosis in particular, nevertheless in some cases the individual components of this combination of stimuli may be used if necessary, for example the physician's voice, relayed through a loudspeaker. All the patients liked this form of suggestion and responded favorably to it. When for some reason the recorded voice could not be transmitted, the patients became upset and made requests for it to be restored. There were some patients, for example U-na with a diagnosis of hysteria, and T-na with a diagnosis of neurasthenia, who thought that this suggestion was

TABLE 1

	Number of observations during stay in hospital									
	Patient K-va					Patient Gr-r				
	In the morning	after dinner	at night	total	%	In the morning	after dinner	at night	total	%
With suggestion:										
Slept	14	9	18	41	85	8	5	15	28	90
Did not sleep	2	3	2	7	15	1	2	—	3	10
Total number of observations	16	12	20	48	100	9	7	15	31	100
Without suggestion:										
Slept	2	7	2	11	19	3	6	4	13	26
Did not sleep	17	16	13	46	81	15	14	8	37	74
Total number of observations	19	23	15	57	100	18	20	12	50	100

so effective that they asked for a copy of the text used, so that they could repeat it to themselves at night at home, as a formula for autosuggestion.

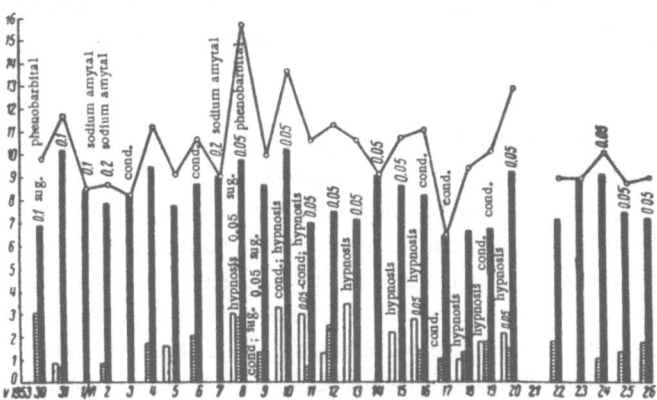

Fig. 16. The effect of hypnosis and sedative drugs on the duration of sleep in P-na. Legend as in Fig. 15. The insufficient duration of sleep on June 11 was due to other causes.

The number of hours of sleep per 24 hours, could be improved when, on the same day, hypnotic suggestion was used in the morning and at other times very small doses of sedative drugs were given, whereas each factor separately often acted less effectively (Fig. 16). We also attempted to investigate the possibility of producing or prolonging sleep by means of the so-called post-hypnotic suggestion, i.e., not immediately after the act of suggestion but after a certain interval of time. This appeared to be quite important, for the physician cannot provide suggestion before the patient goes to sleep each time. Such an investigation was carried out on 14 patients undergoing sleep therapy. Seven of these were suffering from neurasthenia, 4 from hysteria and 3 from neurotic states arising in association with other diseases, notably after encephalitis. In the majority of cases we did not attempt any delayed posthypnotic suggestion to sleep, mainly because we were unable to reach the somnambulistic phase of hypnosis in our patients. Even in patient B-na, who went to sleep quickly and usually did not hear when the doctor left the ward, this type of suggestion was undertaken in only a few isolated instances. The time interval between the suggestion and the anticipated performance—involving for example the period between 10 a.m. and 12 noon—in the majority of cases obliterated all traces of the suggestion and made it more difficult to carry out.

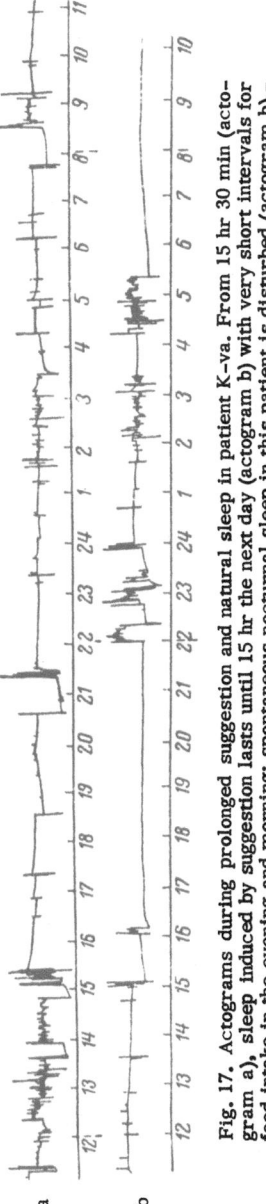

Fig. 17. Actograms during prolonged suggestion and natural sleep in patient K-va. From 15 hr 30 min (actogram a), sleep induced by suggestion lasts until 15 hr the next day (actogram b) with very short intervals for food intake in the evening and morning; spontaneous nocturnal sleep in this patient is disturbed (actogram b)—she goes to sleep at 24 hr, is awake during the night from 2 hr to 3 hr 30 min, and finally awakens at 4 hr 20 min.

In our practice, however, we met individual patients in whom it was easy to induce a somnambulistic state of hypnosis and to suggest going to sleep at a particular time and for any duration. Such patients were Kh-n (case No. 837, 1950), K-va (case No. 148, 1949), and T-t (case No. 48, 1955)[1], all with the diagnosis of hysteria. Prolonged sleep induced in these patients by suggestion alone, without sedative drugs, was recorded by us actographically (Fig. 17).

THE DAILY DURATION OF SLEEP AND ITS CHARACTERISTICS

The majority of authors report very similar figures for the daily duration of drug-induced and conditioned reflex sleep: some report from 12 to 18 hours, others from 14 or even 16 to 20 hours (Druzhinin, Ershov, Kamyanov, Kurilenko, Mukhin, Ostrovskii, Yakovleva, and others). In the majority of our patients (63 out of 79), the mean daily duration of sleep was 10 to 13 hours, and only in a few was it longer, reaching 14 to 15 hours (Table 2).

TABLE 2

Mean daily duration of sleep during treatment (hr and min)	Number of patients
8.00— 8.59	5
9.00— 9.59	6
10.00—10.59	20
11.00—11.59	25
12.00—12.59	18
13.00—13.59	3
14.00—14.59	2
Total	79

When small doses of sedative drugs were given, sleep was possible only if certain favorable conditions prevailed: maximum exclusion of external stimuli (provision of quiet and darkened rooms); the presence of monotonous stimuli; suggestion, etc. In most of these cases the sleep did not give evidence of deep inhibition. A slight noise outside, the least movement in the ward,

[1]Patient of Dr. M. M. Suslova.

the coughing or snoring of one of his neighbors, were sufficient in many cases to awaken the patient or to prevent him from sleeping. After sleep, the patients usually experienced no unpleasant sensations such as vertigo, headache, nausea, etc.

The absence of deep inhibition was confirmed by plethysmographic investigations. In the majority of cases the unconditioned vascular reactions were preserved during the course of treatment, or even appeared in those cases when they were not present before treatment began (Fig. 18).

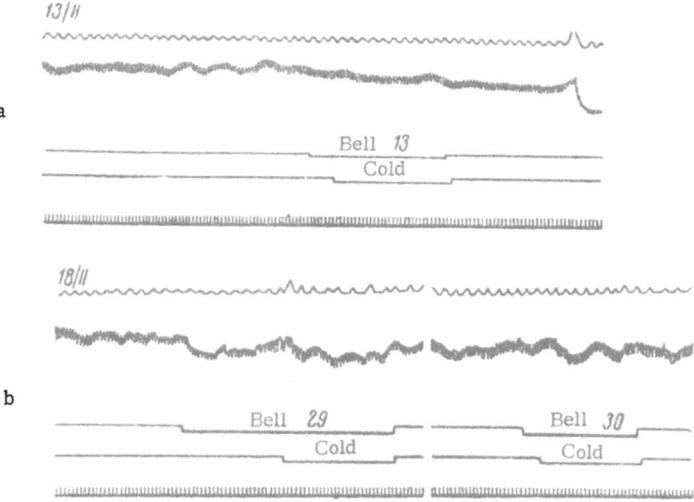

Fig. 18. Plethysmogram of patient L.-na. Significance of the curves, from the top down: respiration, plethysmogram, conditioned stimulus marker, unconditioned stimulus marker, time marker (in seconds). On February 13—before sleep therapy—both conditioned and unconditioned vascular reactions are ill defined. On February 18, in the period of sleep therapy (on the fourth day), the unconditioned reflexes to cold are more pronounced; a conditioned reflex also appears.

On the first day of treatment the duration of sleep was considerably lengthened in patients under the influence of sedative medication, the routine and the environment as a whole. Under these circumstances, as will be shown below, whereas in some patients the regimen and environment are themselves sufficient to prolong sleep considerably (Fig. 19), in the majority of cases sedative drugs play a decisive role. As a test we discontinued sedation in some cases for a day (see Figs. 10 and 11); on that day the curve of duration of sleep fell at once almost to the initial level. It also fell sharply (sometimes below the initial level) on Sundays when the daily administration of drugs was interrupted and patients were visited by relatives. Nocturnal sleep was just as markedly reduced when the sedatives were discontinued as treatment was terminated.

On the curves showing the pattern of sleep duration over several days, we can see considerable fluctuation, in spite of the fact that the same doses of sedative were used and the regimen remained constant. In sleep therapy these fluctuations depend on the influence of different extrinsic and intrinsic disinhibiting stimuli on the cerebral cortex.

There is no doubt that the action of sleep-inducing factors can fully assert itself only when the main stimuli disinhibiting the cortex are removed. These stimuli, and in particular those evoking certain emotions, by creating foci of excitation in the cerebral cortex, may make it more difficult for

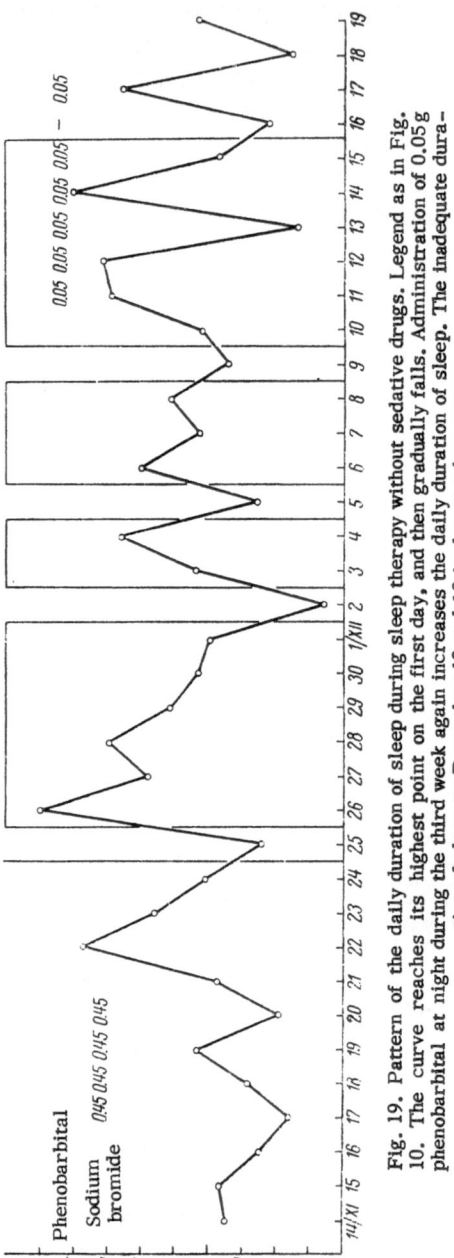

Fig. 19. Pattern of the daily duration of sleep during sleep therapy without sedative drugs. Legend as in Fig. 10. The curve reaches its highest point on the first day, and then gradually falls. Administration of 0.05 g phenobarbital at night during the third week again increases the daily duration of sleep. The inadequate duration of sleep on December 13 and 18 is due to other causes.

Phenobarbital

Sodium bromide

sleep inhibition to develop and tend to counteract the effectiveness of sedative drugs.

Many authors have noted a tendency toward a gradual increase in the duration of sleep in the course of treatment, and have explained this phenomenon by the conditioned reflex influence to the environment as a whole, and to the regimen.

In the majority of cases the pattern of sleep which we observed was different. When the same daily dose of sedative medication was maintained, 19 patients showed a tendency towards a gradual decline in the curve of daily duration of sleep; 14 patients did not display this phenomenon, and only 2 cases showed a gradual rise in the curve. The maximum daily duration of sleep was thus most often found in the first few days of treatment, and especially on the first and second day, after which the curve, in spite of fluctuations, gradually fell. An increase in the sedative dose sometimes prolonged sleep temporarily, but the duration of sleep would again fall off. The simplest explanation of this phenomenon is habituation to the drug. It has, in fact, been shown by direct experiments on animals (Kudryavina, 1954) that with repeated administration of the same dose of sodium amytal to mice, rats, guinea pigs, and rabbits, the duration of sleep falls off.

We made observations on patients in whom sleep therapy was possible without sedative medication, simply by setting up a suitable regimen. Under these conditions the curve of the daily duration of sleep also rose sharply on the first day, and then fell gradually, with fluctuations (see Fig. 19). This is evidently a reflection of the trend of the natural protective sleep inhibition in nervous diseases. As the state of exhaustion of the nervous system is overcome and the working capacity of the nerve cells is restored, the natural protective inhibition begins to weaken, and prolonged sleep yields more and more to wakefulness. The same mechanism evidently also operates in many cases where, in spite of the daily administration of moderate or small doses of sedative, the curve of duration of sleep gradually declines. This view is also confirmed by the fact that, after a break of one day when the patient was awake and, consequently, more fatigued, the curve again rose slightly, and at the end of a week fell once again to even lower levels. In fact it is evident that both these factors are involved, although we attach greater importance to the second. Even the administration of big doses of sedative at the end of the course of treatment has hardly any of the anticipated effect. This phenomenon may, in our opinion, be used as an objective criterion of the weakening of the protective inhibition because of the restoration of the working capacity of the nerve cells, and also as an indication that the treatment is coming to an end.

THE LENGTH OF THE COURSE OF TREATMENT

The duration of treatment in our patients varied on the average between one and three weeks, i.e., between the limits mentioned by the majority of authors. The longer duration of sleep therapy in a small number of cases was due to the severity of their condition. Prolonged courses of treatment were also used during the first years (1949–1951) of our experience with this method. We now think that in some of those cases the duration of treatment could have been shortened, as we more recently do.

As we have said, it is possible to make use of the progressive fall in the duration of sleep, notwithstanding a slight increase in the dose of sedative drugs, as a criterion for the termination of treatment. Another factor of great importance in establishing the individual duration of sleep therapy is how the patient himself feels. After one or two weeks of treatment patients sometimes would say that they are still not sufficiently rested and want to continue sleeping. We usually went along with their wishes, if there were no objective contraindications to the prolongation of sleep therapy. Some patients, however, would say just the opposite. Patient G-va (case No. 267, 1952), for instance, declared after two weeks of sleep therapy that she had slept enough, felt rested, and that her energy and good spirits had returned. Patient F-va (case No. 1077, 1951) declared after three weeks of sleep therapy that she had slept well and did not want to sleep any more. Both patients were discharged as cured.

THE CHANGEOVER FROM SLEEP THERAPY
TO THE ORDINARY ROUTINE

When the administration of sedative drugs is suddenly discontinued at the end of the course of sleep therapy, some patients pass through a period of troublesome insomnia (Fig. 20), when they do not feel quite so well. In view of this fact, in the majority of the later patients, at the end of the course of treatment, we first allowed the evening dose of sedative to be continued, and then we decreased this dose or tried replacing it by placeboes.

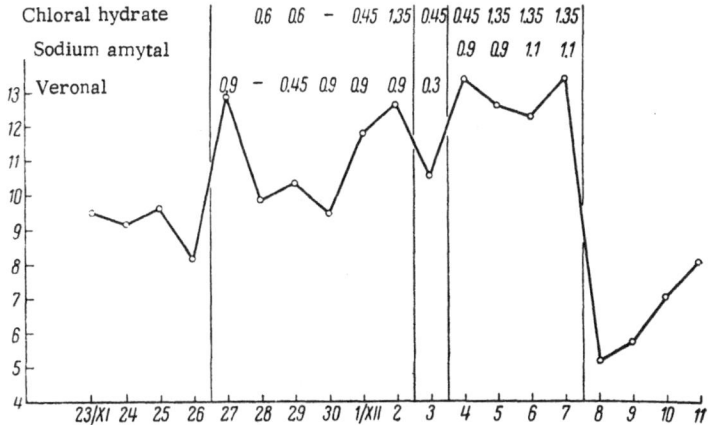

Fig. 20. Pattern of the daily duration of sleep. Legend as in Fig. 10. There is a sharp fall in the curve of the daily duration of sleep on December 8 when sedative drugs were discontinued at the end of the course of sleep therapy.

Le Guillant states that the insomnia which sometimes develops can in one or two days spoil all the good results of the treatment. For this reason he also recommends a gradual decrease in the dosage of sedative drugs.

The next important consideration is the change in the patient's own routine after the end of a course of sleep therapy. Several authors (Davidenkov, Ivanov, Yakovleva, and many others) observe that after sleep therapy is terminated, patients at first feel listless and weak, their moods are unstable and they continue to be troubled by their previous symptoms, and it is only after one or two weeks that improvement supervenes.

After termination of treatment, we observed some traces of general inhibition in our patients, even when small doses of sedative drugs were used. The sudden transition to the ordinary environment may upset the results of treatment, and this did happen in a few cases. Therefore, after we stopped the daily administration of sedatives and the strict enforcement of the sleep regimen, we left the patients free to do as they liked for a few days, and then prescribed additional forms of treatment (physiotherapy, physical training), introduced them to the general life of the hospital and, if necessary, transferred them to the general ward.

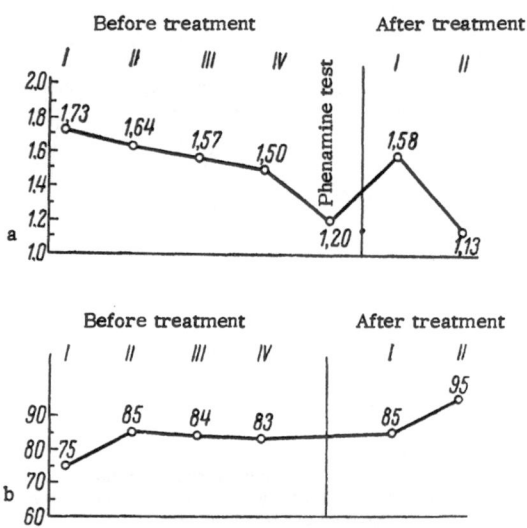

Fig. 21. Pattern of verbal reactions in an association experiment. a) Mean number of disturbed reactions in a group of patients; b) mean percentage reproduction of responses during sleep therapy. The Roman numerals above indicate the serial number of the investigation before and after sleep therapy. The group under the Roman figure I (after treatment) includes investigations made within the first 6 hours after the end of sleep therapy, i.e., when residual manifestations of sleep inhibition are present. Group II includes investigations made during the patient's subsequent stay in hospital (period of improvement).

The results of objective investigation of the higher nervous activity by means of experimental methods (association experiments and plethysmography) show that, for the first few days after sleep therapy, in many cases the state of the higher nervous activity remains stable, or certain of the experimental data may register a slight decline, but progressive improvement is observed after a while. The results of the association experiments show that considerable improvement begins roughly after the second week (Fig. 21). So far as the vascular reflexes are concerned, these often return to normal even later,—according to

of this is the plethysmogram of the patient F-va, in whom the vascular reaction became normal a short time after her discharge from the hospital (Fig. 22).

With patients whose condition is sufficiently serious, it may be desirable to add an additional period of hospital treatment to allow a gradual transition from protective inhibition treatment to the full burden of life, and to consolidate the results achieved.

THE RESULTS OF TREATMENT

To indicate the state of the patient we employed the following terminology: cure, denoting disappearance of the psychiatric symptoms for which the patient was admitted to the hospital, and restoration of fitness for work; considerable improvement, when there was marked improvement, but certain secondary symptoms remained which troubled the patient, but did not significantly affect his fitness for work and general tenor of his life; improvement, when there were definite signs of improvement, with a decreased intensity of the main symptoms although these were not completely abolished; slight improvement; and finally no change.

The results of treatment of the patients (condition at discharge) are summarized in Table 3.

TABLE 3

Results of treatment	Number of patients	%
Cure.................................	15	17.2
Considerable improvement................	32	36.8
Improvement.........................	26	29.9
Slight improvement.....................	11	12.6
No change............................	3	3.5
Total...........	87*	100.0

*The figure given as the total is smaller than the number of patients under our observation (91 patients) because there were four patients whose course of sleep therapy was discontinued.

Cure and improvement were thus observed in 84% of our patients; in 16% there was only slight improvement or no change.

We observed that sleep therapy was of considerable value in the treatment of patients suffering from both neurasthenia and hysteria, but nevertheless we could detect a small difference in this respect between the two groups (Table 4). The number of patients in the column "Improvement and cure" is equally divided between these two forms of neuroses, but in the column "Slight improvement and no change," hysterics account for the greater number of the few patients.

TABLE 4

	Number of patients		
	Improvement and cure	Slight improvement and no change	Total
Neurasthenia.............	31	3	34
Hysteria................	32	7	39*
Total..............	63	10	73

*The number of patients with hysteria here is three less than that given at the beginning of the chapter because of the patients for whom sleep treatment was discontinued (see below).

In analyzing the results of treatment, in relation to the various chief symptoms, we obtained the figures given in Table 5.

TABLE 5

Results of treatment	Number of patients				
	syndrome of anxiety and phobia	astheno-depressive syndrome	syndrome of obsession	hypochon-driacal syndrome	astasia-abasia
Cure................	3	2	—	—	3
Considerable improvement .	6	7	—	—	—
Improvement	7	1	2	—	—
Slight improvement	1	2	1	—	—
No change	1	—	—	2	—
Total...........	18	12	3	2	3

Attention is especially directed to the good results of treatment in three cases of astasia-abasia, and to the failure of treatment in two patients with a hypochondriacal syndrome. Treatment was found to be very effective in syndromes associated with anxiety and also in astheno-depressive syndromes. In obsessional syndromes in three patients we observed fair results, especially when it is remembered that one patient (B-va, case No. 823, 1953), suffering from compulsions, previously discharged as improved, had been twice readmitted to the hospital within a short period because of relapse, and had not been completely relieved of her obsessions.

We next made an analysis of the results of treatment in relation to certain associated diseases, on the basis of which the neurosis had developed. A noteworthy finding is the good results obtained in the treatment of five patients with neuroses associated with hypertension (in the transitory and neurogenic stages). Quite good results were obtained in the treatment of six patients with neuroses developing on a basis of hyperthyroidism. The treatment of neuroses arising in association with other disorders (menopause, concussion, residual manifestations of encephalitis) gave varying results in a small number of patients.

Three patients were discharged without improvement: 1) B-ch (case No. 824, 1950) with a diagnosis of toxic-traumatic encephalopathy with a hypochondriacal syndrome. At follow-up some time afterwards considerable improvement was found to have developed gradually; 2) K-ov (case No. 830, 1950), with neurasthenia of excitable type with a hypochondriacal syndrome. Some improvement was found at follow-up; 3) S-n (case No. 931, 1952), with an hysterical neurosis, a phobic syndrome, and angina pectoris, arising in association with a complicated vocational situation. Improvement followed correction of this situation.

It may be suggested that the lack of improvement in two patients was due to the presence of a hypochondriacal syndrome (which the literature also describes as rather unresponsive to sleep therapy); one of the cases, moreover, was characterized by increased excitation. The third patient had fixated on his unsatisfactory situation, and this prevented the development of an adequate degree of protective inhibition.

Sleep therapy was abandoned in 4 patients because they tolerated it badly: 1) S-n (case No. 849, 1951)—hysteria with a hypochondriacal syndrome; 2) L-na (case No. 172, 1952)—a reactive state following the sudden death of her husband; 3) M-ko (case No. 320, 1953)—hysteria with compulsions (extreme excitation); 4) E-va (case No. 1234, 1951) — hysteria with nausea. Attempts at sleep therapy in the first patient aggravated the hypochondriacal state, and in the second it intensified the reactive experiences. Obviously in both cases the excitation of the pathodynamic foci was caused by positive induction with residual inhibition of part of the cortex. Sleep was discontinued in the third patient on account of her increased excitation, and in the fourth patient because of nausea, which prevented her from taking the sedatives.

FOLLOW-UP

We were able to follow up 27 patients. Three of these were under our observation for only the subsequent few weeks (for two months); the condition of two of them continued good; in the third, improvement occurred only after discharge. We have information on the rest of the patients for longer periods, in some cases four years. Altogether 17 patients were in a satisfactory condition when we examined them. In the patients discharged without reasonable benefit, a gradual improvement took place in all but one.

Relapse of the neurosis developed at various times in 6 patients under the influence of newly developing life difficulties or, in some cases, in association with somatic disease. In three patients, relapse of the neurotic state was associated with serious complicating disease: hypertension in the nephrotic stage, peptic ulcer, and residual postencephalitic manifestations.

Most of the patients who showed improvement, to whom we spoke after their discharge from the clinic, stressed the marked subjective improvement which they had experienced from prolonged sleep.

By way of illustration of the material contained in this book, we will cite two case histories:

Patient S-n[1] (case No. 306), female, aged 41 years, kindergarten teacher, was admitted to the clinic from April 13 to June 3, 1953, because of inability to work, marked irritability, frequent bursts of tears, and intolerance of certain stimuli (noise, bright light)

---

[1]This patient was demonstrated at the Wednesday Clinic on June 17, 1953, to the late Academician K. M. Bykov.

The patient was hypersensitive, emotional, and moody; she sometimes had hypnagogic hallucinations. She had not yet recovered from the severe experiences of the war and blockade and from the loss of her family; everything connected with these memories produced an obvious emotional reaction with tears. The patient was communicative and sociable, and got on well with people. She was oversuggestible under hypnosis.

No organic changes were found in the internal organs and nervous system.

HISTORY. She lived with her mother in poor material circumstances. She did not know her father. She had been left to herself and became reserved in manner. For a few years she was raised in a children's home. Her physical health was not good. From childhood, she had shown artistic tendencies and until recently had been interested in music. She completed seven years of secondary school and industrial training. She worked in a factory. After attending courses of preparatory study at high school, she was accepted at the university. Here she worked very hard, long into the night. Because of domestic difficulties she left the university and started work at the radio center. She did well at this, and was quickly promoted. At first she performed the duties of secretary, and was then transferred to dispatcher. She liked her work and coped successfully with its complexities. She was rather short-tempered and her lack of self-control increased as time went on.

In 1938 the patient was married and gave birth to a child. During the war she continued to work at the radio center. During the bombing and shelling, she tried to suppress her fear and carried on with her usual duties. Later on she became indifferent to danger. She suffered from starvation and malnutrition. During the blockade she gave birth to her second child, but it died a few weeks later. In 1942 the husband and the first child died. The patient was evacuated. She worked as an instructress in a children's home, and completed her training in preschool instruction. In 1949 she began to work in a kindergarten. At times she had to take charge. This made her overtired and nervous. An anxiety state developed and she became more irritable. During an unusually strenuous day she developed an acute hysterical reaction: she screamed, wept, and fell to the ground, and her limbs became limp. From this time on her condition grew worse, and accordingly she was admitted to the clinic.

From the available details we may form the opinion that the process of excitation was quite strong in this patient. Her capacity for work was satisfactory. In spite of her difficult living conditions she had succeeded in obtaining secondary education and had then achieved rapid promotion at work to a responsible position; in wartime, danger had not disturbed her ordinary activity. At the same time, however, she also shows features of a relatively weak nervous system. In childhood, the patient showed asthenic traits and did not enjoy rough company. More recently she could not face up to the demands made on her by her work. She constantly displayed a lack of balance and increased excitability, and these had recently become especially pronounced. So far as mobility is concerned, its satisfactory state is demonstrated by her successful work as a dispatcher in the radio center, and later by her ready adaptation to her enforced evacuation. The emotional character of her reactions and her artistic tendencies suggested that the primary signal system was markedly active.

Investigation of her higher nervous activity by the method of association experiments showed that the mean latent period of the verbal reactions was at the upper limit of normal—2.1 sec. Responses to affectogenic word stimuli were delayed up to 7 or 8 sec and successive inhibition to the next two or three words was observed. In one case there was no reply to the word "family," and in response to the word "war," the patient burst into tears. Perseveration of the replies was only occasionally observed. After administration of 0.01 g phenamine, the mean latent period was considerably shortened and no delays were observed with the responses. These findings indicate the presence of a relatively satisfactory process of excitation and of adequate mobility of the nervous processes. However, the disturbance in verbal reactions to affectogenic word stimuli indicates the presence of pathodynamic foci which play a role in the formation of the neurosis.

A few positive conditioned motor reflexes were formed by the motor-speech method, namely a delaying reflex, differentiation, and conditioned inhibition. The following results were obtained: The latent period of the conditioned motor reactions usually varied between narrow limits: from 0.3 to 0.5 sec, and the magnitude of the motor reflex also was fairly constant. This was evidence of the adequate strength of the process of excitation. Differentiation was developed with regard to position, and now and again was disinhibited (when the patient was "lost in her thoughts"), and on one occasion this led to tears (before the investigation, the patient took part in a conversation which reminded her of her experiences). The delaying reflex and conditioned inhibition were induced with a slight delay. These findings may be regarded as evidence of some degree of weakening of the process of inhibition. The pair of stimuli was altered after the second trial. The patient also completed the task successfully when different positive and negative stimuli were given in turn. This is evidence of satisfactory mobility of the nervous processes in this patient. The verbal response was inexact, which is more often found in patients in whom the primary signal system is dominant.

This patient can be regarded as having a nervous system intermediate in strength and excitable and mobile in type, with predominance of the primary signal system.

CLINICAL DIAGNOSIS: Hysterical neurosis.

The patient was given a course of sleep therapy, lasting from April 21 to May 16. The sedative drug used was phenobarbital, with a maximum daily dose of 0.25 g; suggestion was carried out directly by the physician or by means of a tape recorder; from time to time the sedative was replaced by placeboes. The initial basal level of sleep was 8 to 10 hours a day, and during the course of treatment the daily duration of sleep was maintained at a level of 10 to 14 hours, on some days reaching 16 or 17 hours (Fig. 23).

The patient felt no unpleasant sensations (vertigo, nausea, etc.) indicating incipient toxic manifestations. She felt well and her mood was good for nearly the whole time. She was extremely well disposed toward both the treatment itself and the use of suggestion. During the waking periods we used light remedial gymnastics in bed in order to improve the circulation and respiration, and this also made the patient feel better. At the end of the course of sleep therapy, stimulating psychotherapy was given,

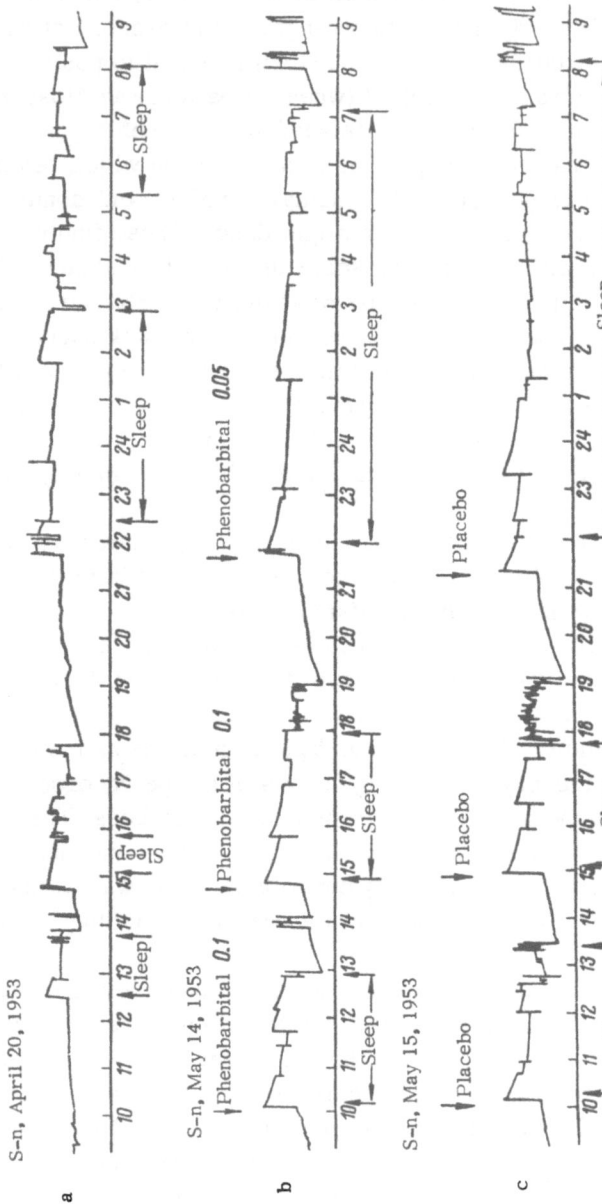

Fig. 23. 24-Hour actograms of patient S-n. a) On the first day that the patient was placed on the therapeutic sleep regimen, no sedative drugs were given; b) at the end of the course of treatment, with phenobarbital given in a daily dose of 0.25 g; c) when placeboes were substituted for the sedatives; the duration of sleep in these instances remained the same as on the previous day.

88

together with hydrotherapy, injections of arsenic and strychnine, bromides, vitamins, and physical exercises.

The patient was eventually discharged much improved. She became more poised and less likely to burst into tears, and her heart stopped bothering her; she was less affected by noise; her state of depression disappeared and she appeared full of life and cheerful, with confidence in her abilities and in her future life prospects.

Further investigation of her higher nervous activity by means of an association experiment now showed a decrease in the mean latent period to 1.3 sec, together with more accurate and composed reactions to affectogenic word stimuli.

FOLLOW-UP. Three years later, the patient is at work and feels well. She refers gratefully to the sleep therapy.

Patient Sm-va (case No. 234), female, aged 32 years, a typist, admitted to the clinic from March 19 to May 12, 1954, because of irritability, frequent bouts of tears, tremors when agitated, weakness, occasional sensations of clouding of the eyes, increased drowsiness, and poor appetite.

The patient was communicative, but depressed in mood, rather slow to respond; she spoke with a quiet voice, but occasionally became irritable; she felt the need for quiet and rest. She showed moderate suggestibility under hypnosis. No organic disturbances of the nervous system were found. Signs of transitory hypertension were present. The blood pressure was 140/90 mm Hg and the pulse rate 84 per minute.

HISTORY. She was born of a working family. In childhood she was modest and shy and avoided large groups of children, staying mainly with her sisters. In her early years at school she studied well, was quiet and disciplined. She was fond of reading. After her fifth year she found her studies more difficult, although she worked hard. When she had to answer in school she became very agitated, trembled, and blushed. After the seventh year of secondary school she attended a pharmaceutical technical school but failed to qualify; she changed to a night school to learn draftsmanship. After completing this course, she started work at a factory as a mechanical draftsman. At the beginning of the war she was evacuated, together with the factory, to the rear. She had a long distance to travel to the factory and had to work very hard; she began to feel tired, but after a short holiday her energies would be revived. On her return to Leningrad, the patient had to contend with many difficulties during the postwar period. She started work as a typist and was given accommodation in the hostel attached to her place of employment. Because of her unsatisfactory living conditions she could not properly keep up with her school studies or obtain proper rest and quiet.

The patient managed to do her job well, in spite of its varied demands and the necessity of living with a large number of people. She had no conflicts at work. She showed impatience only when waiting for transportation; in such circumstances she usually preferred to go on foot. She was never aggressive. She reacted to disagreeable situations with tears. Occasionally she felt drowsy during the day. Not less than 8 hours of sleep was necessary at night for her to regain her energy.

Formerly she had been very sensitive, and would weep at touching passages in a book or at the cinema. Now she had become "quite indifferent."

She was lonely, and was not attracted to the opposite sex. In 1953 hypertension was found, with a maximum blood pressure of 200 mm Hg. Because of the worsening of her general condition, the patient was admitted to the clinic.

From the findings, the process of excitation in this patient could be regarded as fairly weak. Evidence of this is provided by her character during childhood and the asthenic features of her behavior both during her schooldays and at the present time. Nevertheless this patient cannot be classified as belonging to the very weak type for, in spite of the difficulties which she encountered on the way, she took specialized training and until recently worked satisfactorily at her job. The process of inhibition in this patient was considerably weakened, as shown by her impatience and the impossibility of suppressing her emotions. No marked inertia of these processes could be observed in this patient during her life. She coped with changes in her conditions of life, for example during the period of evacuation, and also with the varying demands of her job. At the time of her stay in the hospital, the patient showed a pronounced weakness of nervous processes with the development of manifestations of protective inhibition in the form of severe fatigue and drowsiness, and a need for peace and quiet. No dominance of either signal system was observed.

Upon investigation of the higher nervous activity through association experiments, the latent period of the responses to indifferent word stimuli was found to be increased to 2.2 sec, and disturbed verbal reactions were indicated by the absence of replies, refusals, and delays in response to both affectogenic and indifferent word stimuli; many of the replies showed perseveration, sometimes of many words; also in evidence were emotional reactions, failure to reproduce the original replies, and increased fatigue at the end of the investigation (in the form of lengthening of the latent period). All these findings demonstrate a weakening of both excitatory and inhibitory processes, inertia of these processes and the presence of limiting inhibition, especially strong when affectogenic words were presented.

For a long time it was impossible to develop a conditioned reflex by the motor-speech method, in spite of the use of indirect instruction; difficulties were also encountered in the development of differentiation and conditioned inhibition, and on changing the order of the words—due, we believe, to a lowering of the general tone of the cortex and to the presence of external inhibition from the pathodynamic focus. This was confirmed by the verbal response of the patient before her discharge from the clinic. She attributed the unsatisfactory way in which she had performed the task presented to her before treatment to the fact that she was quite indifferent to it, so that she "didn't understand."

Investigation of respiratory function with the pneumograph showed an arrhythmic type of respiration with frequent deep inspirations, which we interpreted as an indication of disturbance of the vegetative functions. On investigation of the unconditioned vascular reactions with plethysmographic methods, we observed a slightly fluctuating background, with absence of clear reactions to cold and to distant stimuli, which was evidence of the presence of inhibition in higher brain functions. We thus regard the patient as having a strong variant of the weak type of nervous system, with balanced signal systems.

CLINICAL DIAGNOSIS: Neurasthenia (astheno-depressive form).

The patient was treated with sleep therapy. Sodium amytal was used, in a daily dose of 0.3 g, increasing gradually to 0.8 g at the end of treatment. On some days suggestion was given in the morning. After dinner, the patient slept without the aid of sedative drugs. With an initial basal level of daily sleep of 8 to 9 hours, on the first day of the course of treatment the duration of sleep was increased to almost 15 hours (Fig. 24) in spite of the very small dose of sedative drug (0.1 g in the morning and 0.2 g at night); it then began to decrease gradually, with fluctuations. The inclusion of placeboes (keeping a daily dose of 0.1 g sodium amytal) considerably shortened the period of sleep—to 11 hr 40 min per day. On increasing the dose of the sedative to 0.6–0.7 g, the period of sleep was again lengthened to 12 hours or more, although not for long. The course of therapeutic sleep lasted 18 days. During the first few days

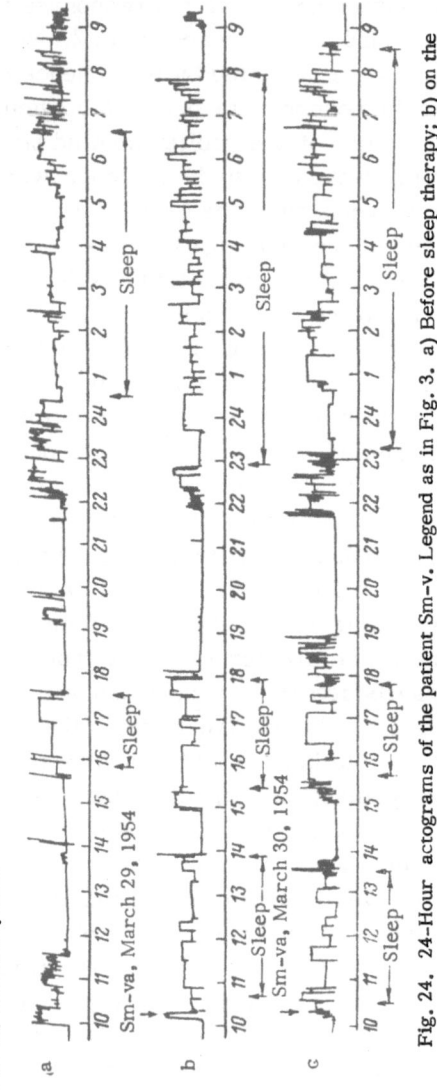

Fig. 24. 24-Hour actograms of the patient Sm-v. Legend as in Fig. 3. a) Before sleep therapy; b) on the first day of treatment; c) on the second day of treatment.

after termination, in spite of the administration of a sedative in the evening, the duration of sleep again fell to the initial level, and then once again gradually rose to 12 hours. Occasional withdrawal of the sedative at night, or its replacement with placeboes, decreased the duration of sleep. During treatment the patient slept gratefully. She felt well, and only occasionally suffered from some nocturnal insomnia; at times tears appeared, but she would control herself. After completion of the course of treatment, the patient noticed that her apathetic state had disappeared, her interest in life had returned, and she began to make plans for the future; now and then she reacted to jokes with laughter, her headaches were much improved, but she still remained irritable, her appetite was poor, and she felt rather weak. Treatment with tonics and sedatives followed: injections of arsenic and strychnine, small doses of bromide with caffeine, vitamins, baths, walks, and remedial gymnastics. The patient's condition continued to improve.

Experimental investigations carried out a few days after the conclusion of sleep therapy gave the following results: In the association experiment the quality of the verbal reactions improved markedly, all the replies were adequate and reproduction was complete. On investigation by the motor-speech method no abnormality could be found. Investigation of the respiratory function a few days after discontinuation of the course of treatment showed that the rate and amplitude were still not sufficiently stable. Before discharge a considerable improvement in the respiratory movements was observed. Upon investigation with the plethysmographic method, unconditioned vascular reflexes began to appear with increasing frequency. The patient was discharged in a greatly improved condition.

CONCLUSION

The material which we have collected provides evidence that sleep therapy is an effective method of treatment for the neuroses, provided, of course, that it is used with proper indications and with suitable technique.

Indications for this treatment are: acute and subacute neuroses and neurotic states with manifestations of exhaustion and asthenia of the nervous system, in which astheno-depressive and phobic syndromes predominate, anxiety and phobic states, and various vegetative visceral disturbances.

In order to gauge the presence of natural protective inhibition and the necessity of restoring the working capacity of the nervous system by prolonged sleep, it may often be possible to make use of certain of the patient's symptoms and complaints, such as intolerance of various stimuli—noise, bright light—the desire of the patient for food, peace and quiet, and his longing for sleep.

The failures sometimes observed after attempts at sleep therapy most often are due to careless selection of patients—for example, when treatment is undertaken with patients who show signs of increased excitation, especially in the motor sphere.

The problem of sleep therapy in patients suffering from obsessions associated with pathological stasis or inertia of the process of excitation (obsessive ideas or compulsions) is still unsolved.

Before a course of treatment is started, preparatory talks should be given to the patients, briefly explaining the nature of neuroses and the importance of Pavlov's method of sleep therapy as being the most humane and rational form of treatment. Patients must be told of the necessity for the special regimen which they must observe throughout the course of treatment. During treatment patients must as far as possible be shielded from external stimuli. In order to avoid excitement patients should not be allowed to keep in touch with their relatives.

For sleep therapy a separate isolated ward is essential, and an isolated department is even better. Experience has shown, however, that the method of sleep therapy can be employed in ordinary hospitals, with the provision of minimal necesary conditions, as well as in specially equipped institutions.

Sleep therapy should not be regarded as a radical method which, if used alone, will completely cure a neurosis. It is rather a particular stage of treatment, to prepare the nervous system for receiving subsequent forms of therapy: training, active psychotherapy and so on; it is therefore important to use it as soon as possible in order to enhance the tone of the nerve cells.

We think that this method of treatment should not become the monopoly of any particular type of hospital or clinic. It may be indicated in various diseases in which there are manifestations of protective inhibition. Sleep therapy should be introduced into a great many hospitals as a definite stage of treatment to be given to certain particular patients,—and not a very wide range.

In the supplement we discuss some problems of the organization and technical equipment of departments for sleep therapy. We hope that this book will help toward the correct evaluation of the Pavlovian method of protective therapy, namely sleep therapy, in the neuroses, and that it will also be useful when this method of treatment is employed in other diseases.

In conclusion I wish to express my deep gratitude to Professors N. A. Kryshova and F. P. Maiorov for their valuable comments and advice during my work on the book.

SUPPLEMENT

TECHNICAL DETAILS FOR THE PROPER
ORGANIZATION OF SLEEP THERAPY

In view of the constantly increasing amount of hospital construction, we think it necessary that advantage should be taken
of our available experience by including special departments for
sleep therapy whenever new hospitals are being planned. For
methods of solving common hygienic and architectural problems,
such as: planning hospitals in the midst of a garden area; building soundproof walls; push-pull ventilation; air conditioning;
systems of radiation heating built in retaining structures (floor,
ceiling, walls), enabling the room to be heated in cold weather
and cooled in hot weather; the construction of window frames;
increasing the area of windows that can be opened to 100% of that
of the frames; the use of special ultraviolet window glass, and
so on—we refer the reader to the article by Yurovskii and Maidanskii (1953). There is no doubt that the fulfilment of all these
technical conditions is especially necessary in departments for
sleep therapy.

Certain other conditions are also required in the organization
of the special department. These include, primarily, the planning
of such a department in a blind end of the building; there must
be no staircases, lifts or other installations which might act as
a source of noise immediately adjoining its walls. Access to the
department should be through a locked door such as is used in
psychiatric departments. Because of the isolated nature of the
department, it must include toilet accommodation, a physiotherapy room with facilities for hydro-, electro-, and photother-
apy, and a dining room,—for which purpose, for the sake of
simplicity, a wide corridor can be adapted. It is desirable to have
cabinets in front of the wards equipped with recording apparatus
(the actograph). It is not advisable to have wash basins on these
cabinets, for the water and waste pipes may act as sources of
unwanted noise.

The corridors must be covered with linoleum to deaden the noise of footsteps.

The optimal size of the ward is evidently one for two patients, but provision must be made of one or two private rooms (for patients who themselves are a source of noise, by coughing, snoring, etc.).

Where a central heating system is in operation the radiators must be fitted with regulators. The electric lighting in the wards must not be too bright nor too dim, for semidarkness may have a depressing effect during waking hours. The corridor (dining room) has to be lighted well enough to permit reading, handicrafts, etc. In addition a blue light (night light) must be used in the wards, the switch being outside the ward.

When the actograph is in use the rubber tubes have to be led along the walls from the beds to the apparatus. For the sake of tidiness of the ward and to avoid accidental damage to or compression of the tubes by movement of furniture, it is advisable to cover the rubber tubes with a metal casing. A connection must be made to the loud-speaker in the ward for transmitting sleep-inducing sound stimuli and recorded suggestion from the tape recorder.

In the construction of the small fountains which act as soporific stimuli, it is necessary to provide on one side (for example, in the toilet accommodation) a water reservoir (like the cisterns in the lavatories, but larger), which fills automatically, and from which water is supplied to the fountains at constant pressure.

The windows of the wards must be provided with dark, movable blinds, and the floor covered with runners and carpets. A cozy atmosphere must be created in the ward. The nurse's office in the corridor must be provided with a signalling system from the ward and a cupboard for the tape recorder.

BIBLIOGRAPHY

SOVIET LITERATURE

Aleksandrova, L. I., and Prokhorova, E. S., "The use of sleep therapy in treatment of nervous diseases." Zhur. Vysshei Nerv. Deyatel. 3, 4 (1953).

Andreev, B. V., "The use of actography in man to study objectively the daily balance between sleep and waking." Byull. Eksptl. Biol. i Med. 3 (1951).

Andreev, B. V., Investigation of Sleep and the Use of Therapeutic Sleep in the Treatment of the Neuroses. Author's abstract of dissertation, Leningrad, 1956.

Asratyan, E. A., "Pavlov's teaching on the protective and remedial role of inhibition and trauma of the nervous system." Nevropatol. i Psikhiat. 4 (1944).

Asratyan, E. A., "The theory and practice of Pavlovian protective-remedial inhibition." Transactions of a Session Commemorating the Tenth Anniversary of the Death of Academician I. P. Pavlov. Izd. AMN SSSR, 1948.

Asratyan, E. A., "The protective and remedial role of the process of inhibition and head injuries." Zhur. Nevropatol. i Psikhait. 54, 1 (1954).

Asratyan, E. A., "The protective and remedial role of inhibition in the spinal cord." Zhur. Vysshei Nerv. Deyatel. 5, 2 (1955).

Baltsvinik, A., " 'Interrupted' therapy." Med. Rabotnik 29, April 26, 1951.

Beilin, P. E., "From pharmacological to physiological sleep." Vrachebnoe Delo 2 (1951)

Bekhterev, V. M., The Therapeutic Value of Hypnotism. St. Petersburg, 1900.

Belousova, M. T., "The syndrome of the obsessional states." Zhur. Nevropatol. i Psikhiat. 54, 11 (1954).

Berdnik, N. G., "The pattern of sleep in patients with neuroses during climatic treatment on the south coast of the Crimea."

Theses on Problems of Inhibition and Sleep Therapy (October, 1955). Tartu, 1955.

Birman, B. N., "Hypnotic suggestion in neuroses and its physiological basis." Arkh. Biol. Nauk SSSR 36, 1 (1934).

Birman, B. N., "The nature and classification of the neuroses in the light of the teaching of Academician I. P. Pavlov." Collection: Soviet Neuropsychiatry, Vol. 2. Leningrad, 1939.

Birman, B. N., "The use of sleep therapy in the treatment of neuroses." Vestnik Akad. Med. Nauk SSSR 5 (1946).

Birman, B. N., "Sleep therapy in the neuroses." Byull. Eksptl. Biol. i Med. 29, 2 (1950).

Birman, B. N., "The role of hypnotic and sleep inhibition in the pathogenesis and treatment of neurotic syndromes." Zhur. Vysshei Nerv. Deyatel. 1, 1 (1951).

Birman, B. N., "The work of I. P. Pavlov in nervous diseases." Nevropatol. i Psikhiat. 20, 6 (1951a).

Birman, B. N., and Vainberg, I. S., "The use of small doses of bromide in the treatment of neuroses." Sovetsk. Vracheb. Gazeta 14 (1935).

Birman, B. N., and Zigel', V. S., "Trial of small doses of bromide in the treatment of neurasthenia." Arkh. Biol. Nauk SSSR 36, Series B, 1 (1934).

Bogachenko, L. S., "Prolongation of sleep in children in the pediatric clinic." Zhur. Vysshei Nerv. Deyatel. 2, 2 (1952).

Bunin, K. V., and Sinitsin, P. D., "Treatment of hypertension by sleep induced by suggestion." Sovet. Med. 10 (1951).

Chalisov, M. A., "Results of the treatment of schizophrenia by prolonged sleep." Transactions of the Central Psychoneurological Institute, Vol. 11, Khar'kov, 1939.

Chukhrienko, D. P., "A therapeutic protective regimen, conditioned reflex sleep therapy, and prolongation of physiological sleep in the practical work of Ukrainian hospitals." Klin. Med. 30, 7 (1952).

Chukhrienko, D. P., "The technique of prolonged, interrupted, conditioned reflex sleep therapy." Khirurgiya 4 (1952a).

Davidenkov, S. N., "The use of sleep therapy in the treatment of nervous diseases." Nevropatol. i Psikhiat. 20, 6 (1951).

Davidenkov, S. N., I. P. Pavlov's Teaching on Neuroses and Their Treatment (stenographic record of lecture). Leningrad, 1952.

Davidenkov, S. N., "Treatment of patients with neuroses in the light of I. P. Pavlov's physiological teaching." Klin. Med. 31, 2 (1953).

Davidenkov, S. N., Clinical Lectures on Nervous Diseases 3, 1957.

Davidenkov, S. N., Dotsenko, S. N., and Yakovleva, M. K., "Treatment of obsessional states with prolonged sleep." Zhur. Navropatol. i Psikhiat. 55, 7 (1955).

Dotsenko, S. N., Obsessional States in Neuroses. Author's abstract of dissertation. Leningrad, 1953.

Druzhinin, A. M., "Treatment of nervous and psychic diseases by fractionated sleep." Zhur. Nevropatol. i Psikhiat. 53, 5 (1953).

Ershov, V. A., "The use of prolonged sleep in the treatment of nervous diseases." Zhur. Nevropatol. i Psikhiat. 54, 11 (1954).

Extended Session of the Presidium of the AMN SSSR with the Ryazan Medical Institute on the Problem: "Experimental and clinical sleep therapy," February 27–28, 1953 (Ryazan). Zhur. Nwvropatol. i Psikhiat. 53, 6 (1953).

Fadeeva, V. K., "Experimental investigation of the cortical dynamics in the manic and depressive phase of cyclothymia." Abstracts of Research Work in Medico-Biological Sciences of the AMN, No. 1, 1947.

Fol'bort, G. V., "Interrelationship between Processes of exhaustion and processes of excitation and inhibition." Conditioned Reflexes. Trud. Ukrain. Psikhonevrol. Inst. 17 (1946).

Gakkel', L. B., The Pathophysiological Mechanism and Clinical Features of the Obsessional Syndrome. Medgiz, 1956.

Galenko, V. E., "New variants of sleep therapy of psychic patients." Zhur. Nevropatol i Psikhiat. 53, 1 (1953).

Gartsshtein, N. G., "Some features and the neurodynamics of cardiazol convulsions." Collected Papers on Neuropsychiatry Commemorating the Jubilee of R. Ya. Golant, Vol. 30, 1940.

Gartsshtein, N. G., "Phasic states in the cerebral cortex of patients with reactive depression." Zhur. Vysshei Nerv. Deyatel. 1, 2 (1951).

Gartsshtein, N. G., "Disturbance of the relationship between the primary and secondary signal systems in reactive depression." Zhur. Vysshei Nerv. Deyatel. 2, 6 (1952).

Gartsshtein, N. G., "The effect of prolonged sleep on the disturbance of the combined working of the signal systems and the associated change in cardiovascular activity in reactive depression." Zhur. Vysshei Nerv. Deyatel. 3, 4 (1953).

Gilyarovskii, V. A., "The psychopathology of prolonged narcosis." Byull. Vsesoyuz. Inst. Eksptl. Med. 3–4 (1936).

Gorodetskaya, S. A., "Experience of sleep therapy treatment." The Teaching of I. P. Pavlov in the Therapeutic Practice of the Psychoneurological Hospital. Moscow, 1954.

Ivanov, G. F., Fundamentals of Normal Human Anatomy, Vol. 2, 1949.

Ivanov, E. S., "Sleep therapy in neuroses, asthenic states, and other disorders of the psychic activity." Zhur. Nevropatol. i Psikhiat. 55, 7 (1955).

Ivanov-Smolenskii, A. G., "Experimental investigations of higher nervous activity in the psychiatric clinic." Byull. Vsesoyuz. Inst. Eksptl. Med. 6–7 (1935).

Ivanov-Smolenskii, A. G., "An experimental and clinical investigation into protective inhibition." Arkh. Biol. Nauk SSSR 12, 1–2 (1936).

Ivanov-Smolenskii, A. G., "The teaching of I. P. Pavlov on protective inhibition and prolonged narcosis in schizophrenia." Transactions of the Second All-Union Congress of Neuropathologists and Psychiatrists 2, 1937.

Ivanov-Smolenskii, A. G., "Prolonged narcosis in schizophrenia and its pathophysiological basis." Arkh. Biol. Nauk SSSR 52, 2 (1938).

Ivanov-Smolenskii, A. G., "Some comparisons between insulin therapy and prolonged narcosis in schizophrenia." Sovetsk. Psikhonevrol. 2 (1939).

Ivanov-Smolenskii, A. G., "The narcotic therapy of schizophrenia." Transactions of the I. P. Pavlov Psychiatric Clinic of the All-Union Institute of Experimental Medicine, Coll. II, Prolonged Narcosis in Schizophrenia (1940).

Ivanov-Smolenskii, The Pathophysiology of Higher Nervous Activity, Moscow, 1949.

Ivanov-Smolenskii, A. G., "Experimental and clinical investigation in the field of protective inhibition and prolonged therapeutic sleep." Zhur. Vysshei Nerv. Deyatel. 1, 3 (1951).

Ivanov-Smolenskii, A. G., "General functional disturbances of higher nervous activity and the pathodynamic structures in neuroses and reactive states." Trudy Inst. Vysshei Nerv. Deyatel., Ser. Patofiziol. 1 (1955).

Kamyanov, I. M., "The therapeutic use of conditioned reflex sleep." Voenno-Med. Zhur. 2 (1952).

Kerbikov, O. V., Zorina, E. S., and Il'inskii, Yu. A., "Prolonged sleep therapy by administration of solutions containing alcohol by intravenous drip." Nevropatol. i Psikhiat. 20, 4 (1951).

Kokin, M. K., Antroptseva, L. A., and Plavinskaya, V. V., "The combined treatment of certain forms of psychic diseases by prolonged sleep and thiamin." Vrachebnoe Delo 8 (1951).

Kondratenko, O. I., "Treatment of patients with writer's cramp by prolonged, interrupted sleep." Zhur. Nevropatol. i Psikhiat. 53, 1 (1953).

Konstantinov, V. A., "Prolongation of survival of white mice in a hermetically sealed vessel. Communication 2. The influence of narcosis at various external temperatures." Collection: Mechanisms of Pathological Reactions, 11–15, 1949.

Kudryavina, N. A., "The course of artificial sleep induced by sodium amytal." Farmakol. i Toksikol. 2 (1954).

Kurilenko, P. S., "The sleep therapy of certain diseases." Voenno-Med. Zhur. 10 (1952).

Landkof, B. L., "Prolonged sleep therapy in psychiatric practice." Problems of the Pathophysiology and Therapy of Schizophrenia, GMI Ukrainian SSR, 1938.

Levina, Ts. A., and Terletskaya, T. M., "Sleep therapy without drugs in hypertension and other internal diseases." Sovet. Med. 10 (1951).

Lizunova, M. I., "Treatment of hypertension by prolonged sleep." (Kuibyshev). Klin. Med. 9 (1950).

Lukina, A. M., "The technique of sleep therapy (psychoses and neuroses)." Zhur. Nevropat. i Psikhiat. 53, 4 (1953).

Maiorov, F. P., "Hysteria in a strong type of nervous system." Proceedings of a Conference on Problems of Psychogenia, Psychotherapy and Mental Hygiene, Leningrad, 1946.

Mukhin, V. M., "Prolonged sleep therapy in patients with neurotic conditions." Voenno-Med. Zhur. 10 (1953).

Myasishchev, V. N., "The pathogenesis of the neuroses." Zhur. Nevropatol. i Psikhiat. 55, 7 (1955).

Narbutovich, I. O., and Golovina, V. P., "The action of alcohol in schizophrenia." Arkh. Biol. Nauk SSSR 36, 1 (1934).

Narbutovich, I. O., and Povorinskii, Yu. A., "The use of combined insulin and narcotic therapy in schizophrenia." Transactions of the Ukrainian Central Psychoneurological Institute (Treatment of Schizophrenia), Vol. 2, 1939.

Naumova, V. V., "The action of certain hypnotics on schizophrenic patients." Transactions of the 14th Session of the Ukrainian Psychoneurological Institute, Vol. 23, 1947.

Nikulin, K. G., "The clinical importance of conditioned reflex reactions." Klin. Med. 9 (1951).

Obnorskii, P. P., "Organization of the hospital on the basis of I. P. Pavlov's teaching." Sovet. Zdravookhr. 1 (1952).

Ostrovskii, M. I., "Sleep therapy in certain diseases of the nervous system." Voenno-Med. Zhur. 10 (1953).

Ozeretskovskii, D. S., Obsessional States. Moscow,. 1950.

Pavlov, I. P., "The tentative excursion of a physiologist into the field of psychiatry." Complete Collected Works, Vol. 3, 1949.

Pavlov, I. P., "The physiology of higher nervous activity." Complete Collected Works, Vol. 3, 1949a.

Pavlov, I. P., "An attempted physiological explanation of the symptomatology of hysteria." Complete Collected Works, Vol. 3, 1949b.

Pavlov, I. P., "An attempted physiological explanation of the obsessional neurosis and of paranoia." Complete Collected Works, Vol. 3, 1949c.

Pavlov's Wednesdays, Vols. 1 and 2, 1949.

Pavlov's Wednesday Clinics, Vol. 1, 1954.

Pervov, L. G., Study of the Higher Nervous Activity in Patients with Hysteria. Author's abstract of dissertation. Leningrad, 1957.

Petrova, M. K., Latest Data on the Mechanism of Action of Bromides on the Higher Nervous Activity and on Their Therapeutic Use, on Experimental Grounds. Moscow, 1935.

Petrova, M. K., "A series of castrated dogs with different types of nervous system, at even later periods after castration.

(Two cases of abortive catatonia)." Trudy Fiziol. Lab. I. P. Pavlova 7 (1937).

Petrova, M. K., "Narcotic and hypnotic sleep inhibition and their therapeutic value in experimental neurotic dogs." Fiziol. Zhur. SSSR 1 (1946).

Platonov, K. I., "The importance of hypnoid phases of the cerebral cortex in the genesis and therapy of neurotic states." Transactions of the 14th Session of the Ukrainian Psychoneurological Institute, Vol. 23, 1947.

Platonov, K. I., "The study of the importance of hypnotic sleep inhibition as a therapeutic measure in certain pathological conditions in man." Zhur. Vysshei Nerv. Deyatel. 2, 3 (1952).

Povorinskii, Y. A., "Combined treatment of patients with schizophrenia by sleep and insulin." Zhur. Nevropatol. i Psikhiat. 53, 1 (1953).

Popov, A. K., "The study of sleep in man by the method of actography." Zhur. Vysshei Nerv. Deyatel. 4, 1 (1954).

Propp, M. V., Changes in the Vascular Conditioned and Unconditioned Reflexes in Functional and Organic Diseases of the Central Nervous System. Author's abstract of dissertation, Leningrad, 1953.

Protopopov, V. P., "Principles and methods of protective therapy." Transactions of the 2nd All-Union Congress of Neuropathologists and Psychiatrists, 2. Moscow, 1937.

Rakhlin, A. V., "Treatment of gastric and duodenal ulcer by prolonged sleep." Sovet. Med. 10 (1948).

Rashkovan, M. A., "Treatment by protective remedial inhibition in the neurological department of the hospital." Voenno-Med. Zhur. 10 (1951).

Rasin, S. D., and Vernikova, R. A., "The use of 'electrosleep' and conditioned reflex sleep in psychic patients." Vrachebnoe Delo, 5 (1952).

Rikhter, G. E., "Treatment of schizophrenia by prolonged narcotic sleep." Arkh. Biol. Nauk SSSR 47, 2 (1937).

Rikhter, G. E., "Prolonged interrupted sleep as a pathogenetic method of treatment of schizophrenia." Collected papers by neuropathologists and psychiatrists of the Latvian SSR. Neuropathology and Psychiatry. Izd. AN Latvian SSR, Riga, 1956.

Rozhnov, V. E., "The effectiveness of therapeutic suggestion in prolonged hypnotic sleep." Zhur. Nevropatol. i Psikhiat. 53, 6 (1953).

Sennikov, I. O., "Characteristics of the electrolytes of the protein fractions of the blood and the blood sugar in the treatment of neuroses by prolonged sleep." Collected papers by neuro-pathologists and psychiatrists of the Latvian SSR. Neuropathology and Psychiatry. Izd. AN Latvian SSR, Riga, 1956.

Seredina, M. I., "Experimental investigation of the neurodynamics of the convulsive fit in epileptic children." Proceedings of the 9th Conference on Physiological Problems, 1941.

Seredina, M. I., "Pathogenetically based treatment of neurosis in obsessional states." Trudy Inst. Vysshei Nerv. Deyatel., Ser. Patofiziol. 1 (1955).

Sereiskii, M. Ya., "Treatment of schizophrenia by prolonged sleep." Sovet. Med. 5 (1937).

Sereiskii, M. Ya., Zeleva, M. S., and Lando, L. I., "Treatment of patients with schizophrenia by prolonged sleep." Zhur. Nevropatol. i Psikhiat. 53, 10 (1953).

Shchelovanov, N. M., "The ontogenesis of waking and sleep in the infant." Proceedings of Extended Scientific Committees of the AMN SSSR on the Experimental Basis of Sleep Therapy. Moscow, 1954.

Shevelev, N. A., "Prolonged narcosis in the treatment of psychoses." Sovet. Psikhonevrol. 2 (1936).

Shoshin, B. G., "Experience of conditioned reflex sleep in a disturbed part of a psychoneurological hospital." The Teaching of I. P. Pavlov in Psychoneurological Therapeutic Practice. Moscow, 1954.

Shpak, V. M., "The treatment of pre-senile psychoses by prolonged interrupted sleep combined with biogenic stimulators." Zhur. Vyssh. Nerv. Deyatel. 52, 8 (1952).

Shpak, V. M., "The use of physiological mechanisms of prolonged sleep in the treatment of neuroses and some psychoses." Zhur. Vysshei Nerv. Deyatel. 3, 4 (1953).

Shpir, R., "The treatment of schizophrenia by prolonged sleep." Transactions of the Central Psychoneurological Institute, Vol. 11. Khar'kov, 1939.

NON-SOVIET LITERATURE

Beaunis, H., Hypnotism, St. Petersburg, 1889. [Russian translation.]

Forel, A., Hypnotism or Suggestion and Psychotherapy. Leningrad, 1928. [Russian translation.]

Grasset, J., L'Hypnotisme et la Suggestion. Paris, 1903.

Hesse, Baumgart u. Dickmann. Zur Wirkungssteigerung der Schlafmittel durch Analgetica. Klin. Wchnschr. 11, 1932.

Johnson, H. M., and Swan, T. H., Sleep. Psychol. Bull. 27, 1 1930.

LeGuillant, L., La conduite de la cure de sommeil chez les malades mentaux. La Raison, N. 6, 1953.

Liébeault. Du sommeil et des états analogues considérés surtout au point de vue de l'action moral sur la physique. Paris, 1866.

Löwenfeld, Hypnotism and Its Technique, Khar'kov, 1928. [Russian translation.]

Moll, A., Der Hypnotismus. Berlin, 1924.

Sapir, M. and Levy, M., Quelques remarques sur la cure de sommeil. La Raison, N. 6, 1953.

Szymanski, J. S., Eine Methode zur Untersuchung der Ruhe und Aktivitätsperioden bei Tieren. Arch. f. d. g. Physiol., 158, 1914.

Szymanski, J. S., Aktivität und Ruhe bei den Menschen. Ztschr. f. angew. Psychol. 20, 1922.

Vogt, O., Ueber die Natur der Suggestion und Hypnose. Ztschr. f. Hypnot., 1895.

Wetterstrand, O., Der Hypnotismus und seine Anwendung in der praktischen Medicin. Wien, 1891.

SUPPLEMENTARY BIBLIOGRAPHY

(Compiled by Dr. Joseph Wortis)

Arch. Phys. Ther. 9, 1 (1957).

Arian, E., "La cura conit sonno indotto da alcool etilico: metodo ed indicazioni." Nevrasse 5, 643 (1955).

Azima, H., "Prolonged sleep treatment in mental disorders: some new psychopharmacological considerations," J. Ment. Sc. 101, 593 (1955).

Azima, H., "Sleep treatment in mental disorders; results of four years of trial," Dis. Nerv. Syst. 19, 523 (1958).

Baumann, R., Physiologie des Schlafes und Klinik der Schlaftherapie, VEB Verlag Volk und Gesundheit, Berlin, 1953, 227 pp.

Bollinger, H., "Beitrag zur Beurteilung der Erfolgsaussichten von Schizophreniebehandlungen nach Dauernarkosen," Psychiatria 135, 211 (1958).

Cameron, D. E., and Pande, S. K., "Treatment of chronic paranoid schizophrenic patient, "Canad. M.A.J. 78, 92 (1958).

"Les cures de sommeil, deux methodes actuelles en France," Sem. méd. profes. 33, 1710 (1957).

Demant, E., "Der Schlaf als Heilschlaf in der antiken und heutigen Medizin," Arch. Phys. Ther. 9, 9 (1957).

Diury, P., Bobon, J., and Collard, J., "Considérations sur les cures de sommeil potentialisees et les cures neuroleptiques en psychiatrie," Act. Neurol. Psychiat. Belg. 57, 185 (1957).

Diury, P., Bobon, J., and Collard, J., "L'hypnothérapie clinique et la chemiothérapie hypothermisante," Rev. med. Liege 13, 209 (1958).

Ey, H., and Faure, H., "Sleep therapy and the use of chlorpromazine," Internat. Rec. Med. 170, 1 (1957).

Ferraro, A., Roisin, L., Capone, P., and Stein, N. E., "A new method of treatment of affective psychoses and psychoses with depressive features," J. Nerv. Ment. Dis. 111, 271 (1950).

Giljarowski, W. A., Elektroschlaf, Verlag Volk und Gesundheit, Berlin, 1956.

Habs, H., "Neue Möglichkeiten der subkortikalen Schutzhemmungstherapie," Zts. ges. inn. Med. 12, 1123 (1957).

Harrer, G., "Möglichkeiten, Ziele und Grenzen der Schlaftherapie," Wien. klin. Wschr. 69, 109 (1957).

Ivanov, V., "Le traitement de certaines psychoses par le sommeil de longue durée et interrompu," Psychiatria 136, 380 (1958).

Ivanov-Smolenskii, A. G., Essays on the Patho-Physiology of the Higher Nervous Activity, Foreign Languages Publishing House, Moscow, 1954, 349 pp.

Jeri, R., "Accidentes fatales durante el tratamiento por electronarcosis," Rev. Neuro-Psiquiat. 20, 30 (1957).

Kerbikov, O. V., "Treatment of mental disease by sleep," Lancet 1, 744 (1955).

Kläsi, J., "Über die therapeutische Anwendung der Dauernarkose mittels Somnifen bei Schizophrenen," Z. Ges. Neurol. Psychiat. 74, 557 (1922).

Kleinsorge, H., and Rösner, K., "Schlaftherapie mit Phenothiazinderivaten," Ther. Gegenwart 95, 441 (1956).

Kleinsorge, H., Rösner, K., and Dressler, S., "Experimentelle Untersuchungen über den Elektroschlaf," Arch. Phys. Ther. 9, 20 (1957).

Labhardt, F., Betrachtungen zur Schlafbehandlung in der Phychiatrie und psychosomatischen Medizin," Schweiz. Arch. Neurol. Psychiat. 84, 341 (1959).

Laboucarie, J., and Combes, P., "Valeur et limites des cures de sommeil en psychiatrie," Toulouse méd. 55, 221 (1954).

Lienau, C., "Heilschlafbehandlung mit Pacatal bei Alkoholismus und Morphinismus," Münch. Med. Wschr. 99, 80 (1957).

Martini, F., "La terapia del sonno nella practica psichiatrica; risultati ottenuti in un gruppo di 111 malati," Riv. pat. nerv. ment. 77 549 (1956).

Martini, F., and Giagiotti, F., "Esplorazione della personalita in 50 schizofrenici trattati con la terapia del sonno," Riv. pat. nerv. ment. 78, 1095 (1957).

Monnerot, E., Puech, J., Benichou, L., Robin, C., and Langlois, H., "La cure de sommeil conserve-t-elle des indications psychiatriques? Considérations personnelles portant sur 700 cas," Ann. Méd.-Psychol. 115, 845 (1957).

Monro, A. B., "Electronarcosis in the treatment of schizophrenia," J. Ment. Sc. 106, 254 (1950).

Moore, D., "The use of sleep therapy in psychiatric treatments," Med. J. Austral. 45, 9 (1958).

Moreau, P. J., "Réflexions sur des échecs de la cure de sommeil dans la mélancolie," Méd. Lyon 38, 407 (1957).

Norry, J. T., Terapeutica por el Sueño Prolongado, Editorial Alfa Buenos Aires, 1953, 326 pp.

Palmer, H. A., "The value of continuous narcosis in the treatment of mental disorder," J. Ment. Sc. 83, 636 (1937).

Parfitt, D. N., "A comparison of prolonged narcosis and convulsion therapy in mental disorder," J. Ment. Sc. 92, 128 (1946).

Patterson, A. S., and Milligan, W. L., "The technique and application of electronarcosis," Proc. R. Soc. Med. 41, 575 (1948).

Pavlov, I. P., Lectures on Conditioned Reflexes, translated by W. Horsley Gantt, International Publishers, New York, 1928, 414 pp.

Pavlov, I. P., Conditioned Reflexes and Psychiatry, translated by W. Horsley Gantt, International Publishers, New York, 1941, 199 pp.

Pavlov, I. P., Selected Works, Foreign Languages Publishing House, Moscow, 1955, 654 pp.

Piazzesi, W., "Considerazioni e dati sulla ipnoterapia in campo psichiatrico," Rev. patol. nerv. ment. 75, 541 (1954).

Pfeil, K., Neue Wege in der Heilschlaftherapie; Erfahrungen bei Kombinationen verschiedener Phenothiazinderivate," Medizinische, No. 13, 463 (1957).

Puech, J., and Robin, C., "Étude comparative des effets de la cure de sommeil medicamenteux et de la chlorpromazine injectable dans les psychoses," Sem hôp. 32, 3252 (1956). La Raison: Revue bimenstruelle, No. 6, July, 1953.

Raymond, M. J., Lucas, C. J., Beesley, M. L., and O'Connell, B. A., "A trial of five tranquillizing drugs in psychoneurosis," Brit. M. J., No. 5036, 63 (1957).

Rees, L., "Electronarcosis in treatment of schizophrenia," J. Ment. Sc. 95, 625 (1949).

Rees, L., "A comparative study of the value of insulin coma, electronarcosis, electroshock and leucotomy in treatment of schizophrenia," Int. Psychiat. Congress Proc. 4, 303. Herman et Cie, Paris, 1952.

Reichlin, S., Koussa, M. G., and Witt, F. W., "Effect of prolonged sleep therapy and of chlorpromazine on plasma protein-bound iodine concentration and plasma thyroxine turnover," J. Clin. Endocrin. 19, 692 (1959).

Rogers, J., Toga, M., Mouren, P., and Gastaut, H., "Constatations anatomiques dans un cas d'épilepsie du sevrage après cure de sommeil," Rev. Neurol. 100, 741 (1959).

Rosman, N. P., "Prolonged sleep therapy in the treatment of mental disorders," McGill M. J. 27, 45 (1958).

Sargant, W., and Slater, E., Physical Methods of Treatment in Psychiatry, E. & S. Livingstone, Ltd., Edinburgh and London, 1956, 351 pp.

Schmidt, E., "Erfahrungen mit der Schlaftherapie, insbesondere bei nervösen Erschöpfungszuständen und Neurosen," Med. Klin. 52, 1267 (1957).

Semadeni, G., and Tchicaloff, M., "L'électro-sommeil," Méd. et Hyg. 15, 123 (1957).

Steiner, U., "Über das EEG bei Neurosen unter Berucksichtigung der Schlaftherapie," Psychiat. Neurol. med. Psychol. 10, 25 (1958).

Walsh, J., "Continuous narcosis: the advantages of oral somnifaine," J. Ment. Sc. 93, 255 (1947).

Weidner, K., "Die Theorie des Zweiphasenheilschlaf," Deutsch Med. J. 10, 343 (1959).

Weir Mitchell, S., Fat and Blood, 4th Ed., Lippincott, 1885.

Wortis, J., Soviet Psychiatry, Williams and Wilkins, Baltimore, 1950, 314 pp.